AF412026

FROM HIPPOCRATES TO VIRCHOW
Reflections on Human Disease

L ife is short, and Art long; the crisis fleeting; experiment perilous, and decision difficult. The physician must not only be prepared to do what is right himself, but also to make the patient, the attendants, and the externals cooperate.

—Hippocrates: *Aphorisms* I.1.

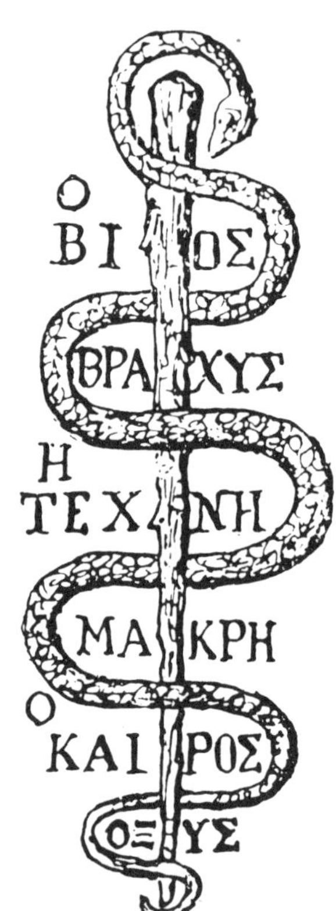

FROM HIPPOCRATES TO VIRCHOW

◆ ◆ ◆ ◆ ◆ ◆ ◆ ◆ ◆ ◆ ◆ ◆

Reflections on Human Disease

James M. Byers, MD
Associate Professor of Pathology
University of Arizona College of Medicine
Tucson, Arizona

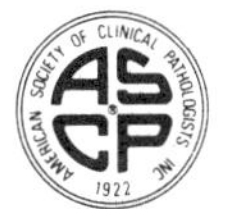

ASCP Press ◆ American Society of Clinical Pathologists ◆ Chicago

Jacket illustration:
Courtesy of the Bettmann Archive, New York

Library of Congress Cataloging-in-Publication Data

Byers, James M., 1944–
  From Hippocrates to Virchow.

  Bibliography: p.
  Includes index.
  1. Pathology—History. I. Title.
RB15.B94 1987   616.07'09   87–18835
ISBN 0–89189–257–5

Printed in the United States of America.

92 91 90 89 88   5 4 3 2 1

This book is dedicated to Greenfield, Ohio's, beloved Dr. Marty, who, by his very hand, with kindness, care, and love for his patients, led me into the world and ways of medicine.

Contents

Foreword

Some years ago, in times we are prone now to think of as simpler, when rustic metaphors were more appropriately current and farm-boy similes and anecdotes were effective means of relating biomedical concepts to the prior experiences of medical students, my advisor at a small midwestern college was wont to admonish us for failure to keep up our extracurricular reading, particularly of classical literature. One evening at a meeting of the premed club he was particularly insistent until one of my classmates rebutted, "Dr. Stevens, when you are in the middle of a pasture with an angry bull, you don't stop to pick daisies."

In a couple of senses, this little book may be a daisy.

The premedical and medical students of today, surrounded by the constantly expanding kaleidoscope of science, feel even more pursued, although they might be more inclined to refer to eighteen-wheelers than to rutting cattle. Nevertheless, I have a conviction that they, as well as the generation before them, harbor a repressed interest in the stories and histories of medicine before their day. Dr. Byers is undoubtedly correct in his introductory emphasis on the importance of physicians giving consideration to the truly basic components of their education as professionals, but I hope sincerely that his estimate of the solitary eminence of the oath of Hippocrates in their experience is descriptive of only a short segment of their careers.

There are several books in my library that have survived my moves from university to university and city to city, while once frequently referenced texts have been abandoned or supplanted. Willius and Keys' *Cardiac Classics* and Long's *Readings in Pathology* were book prizes of one sort or another; Osler's *Aequanimitas* was an altruistic gift from a drug house to me as well as to every other graduate of that time. These volumes have been useful in the preparation of lectures and the writing of manuscripts, for leisure reading, and even for the pleasure of knowing that I possessed their contents when I read a reference to them in someone else's writing. Although Dr. Byers compiled his little book for second-year medical students, it will be a valuable addition to the library of any thoughtful physician or other educated person who is, or should be, concerned with the historical perspective of western thought regarding the issues of medicine and society.

Also a long occupant of shelf space in my home—and I know the situation is similar for several colleagues, and I suspect it is so for many others—has been a set of the Encyclopaedia Britannica's *Great Books of the Western World,* filled with readings waiting for years for me to develop the initiative, or find the time, to take advantage of their presence. Under Dr. Byers' guidance, it has been a pleasure to be led into the numerous topics under which he classifies his selections and comments and to find that they have incited in me a desire to read further in the references and find out more about the thoughts from which a particular quotation is derived.

I suspect other readers will find, as did I, that on occasion an assigned association of a given quotation seemed imaginative, if not fanciful, particularly with consideration of the larger text discovered on turning to the reference; but I cannot fault Dr. Byers for I am sure the pleasure of such argument would carry me into similar disagreement with the classification of any other editor. It is the stimulus of recognition of partially familiar things that leads a reader to wonder whether classical authors were dealing with entities as we know them and that excites the imagination as to just what diseases had been experienced. Inevitably, we will have different insights into such partial and incomplete databases; but, until all writings are stored in larger and larger computers instead of books, and programs of artificial intelligence erase all possibilities of individual interpretations, there will be a joy in consulting ancient wisdom.

The five headings chosen by Dr. Byers for his

selections and comments guide one most helpfully in pursuing an interest, but the index will be even more appreciated by inquisitive readers and potential authors looking for an appropriate allusion. Look under "leprosy," read the thought of the humor that affects the color of hair, and consider modern ideas of why hair appears white even without the loss of all pigment. Perhaps Grecian Formula has better claim to the antiquity in its name than I ever imagined!

The relation to *Great Books* makes this potentially an everyman's guide to relevant classical literature and will inspire us to seek access to the other references utilized by Dr. Byers.

David E. Smith, MD
Galveston, Texas

REFERENCES

Long ER: *Selected Readings in Pathology from Hippocrates to Virchow.* Springfield, Ill: Charles C. Thomas, 1929.

Osler W: *Aequanimitas; with other Addresses to Medical Students, Nurses and Practitioners of Medicine,* ed 3. Philadelphia: Blakiston Co, 1932.

Willius FA, Keys TE: *Cardiac Classics.* St. Louis: CV Mosby Co, 1941.

Introduction

The medical students at the University of Arizona College of Medicine traditionally recite an amended version of the Hippocratic oath at their collegial convocation just before commencement. It has occurred to me over the years that for many of the graduating class this was perhaps their first and last conscious contact with this concentrated expression of what physicians very early on in the history of western medicine learned about professionalism in medicine, respect for patients, good medical manners, and the importance of considering the whole patient in the broader context of life and society.

Of late, it has become more and more important for physicians to step back, pause a while, and ponder what it takes to make a person into a suitably educated member of the medical profession. There is so much information to process, and the time is so scarce!

Our medical colleges properly concentrate on basic medical sciences, pathophysiology, mechanisms of disease, diagnosis, prognosis, and the psychosocial aspects of modern medical practice; but so often the students I have known have gone through their vigorous, achievement-oriented curriculum without even pausing to think about, much less reflect upon, the history of what they are getting into and how the profession has evolved in various contexts over the past 25 or so centuries. Many of today's dilemmas, problems, and difficulties thought by many to be reflections of twentieth-century information overload, corporate medicine, or litigious health consumers are *not at all new phenomena*. They have been present from time immemorial and are but an aspect of one of the most difficult of human tasks—caring for, in a personal and intimate way, and trying to cure a frightened person whose life has had a major disruption, a person likely to be disoriented and dysphoric—an acutely ill human being.

Philosophers, physicians, theologians, literary artists, and medical scientists have all contributed to our current perspective on human illness and disease. The extracts from great literary works assembled here demonstrate for us some of the most important and persevering insights into the relationship between man and nature. In this work the included descriptions and discussions about the hurt and the healer, the disoriented and the doctor date back centuries, but most are still relevant to current medical practice.

Many of the works herein quoted are rather well-known by author or title, even commonly alluded to in a general sense; some concepts inferentially derived from them are discussed in classrooms and on ward rounds; but today's students and practitioners rarely read the actual words. While most of the ideas are in some way expressed in twentieth-century medicine, the precise origins remain to most, obscure. This work is an attempt to bring these important, relevant ideas into the conscious mind of today's students of medicine, to help those in our profession better appreciate the context from which it arose.

The study of human disorders and diseases continues to evolve; definitions change, structural classifications (like molecules) rearrange, functional measurements become more precise and accurate, and our understanding of human biology advances; yet the medical doctor and his or her patient still have to face the unknown and come to an accommodation with medicine and each other together. Somehow, it seems that the wisdom of the ages ought to make their joint effort less painful, perhaps more comfortable, and, one would hope, more satisfying.

The Hippocratic Oath

I swear by Apollo the physician, by Aesculapius, Hygeia, and Panacea, and I take to witness all the gods, all the goddesses, to keep according to my ability and my judgment the following Oath:

To consider dear to me as my parents him who taught me this art; to live in common with him and if necessary to share my goods with him; to look upon his children as my own brothers, to teach them this art if they so desire without fee or written promise; to impart to my sons and the sons of the master who taught me and the disciples who have enrolled themselves and have agreed to the rules of the profession, but to these alone, the precepts and the instruction. I will prescribe regimen for the good of my patients according to my ability and my judgment and never do harm to anyone. To please no one will I prescribe a deadly drug, nor give advice which may cause his death. Nor will I give a woman a pessary to procure abortion. But I will preserve the purity of my life and my art. I will not cut for stone, even for patients in whom the disease is manifest; I will leave this operation to be performed by practitioners (specialists in this art). In every house where I come I will enter only for the good of my patients, keeping myself far from all intentional ill-doing and all seduction, and especially from the pleasures of love with women or with men, be they free or slaves. All that may come to my knowledge in the exercise of my profession or outside of my profession or in daily commerce with men, which ought not to be spread abroad, I will keep secret and will never reveal. If I keep this oath faithfully, may I enjoy my life and practice my art, respected by all men and in all times; but if I swerve from it or violate it, may the reverse be my lot.

FROM HIPPOCRATES TO VIRCHOW
Reflections on Human Disease

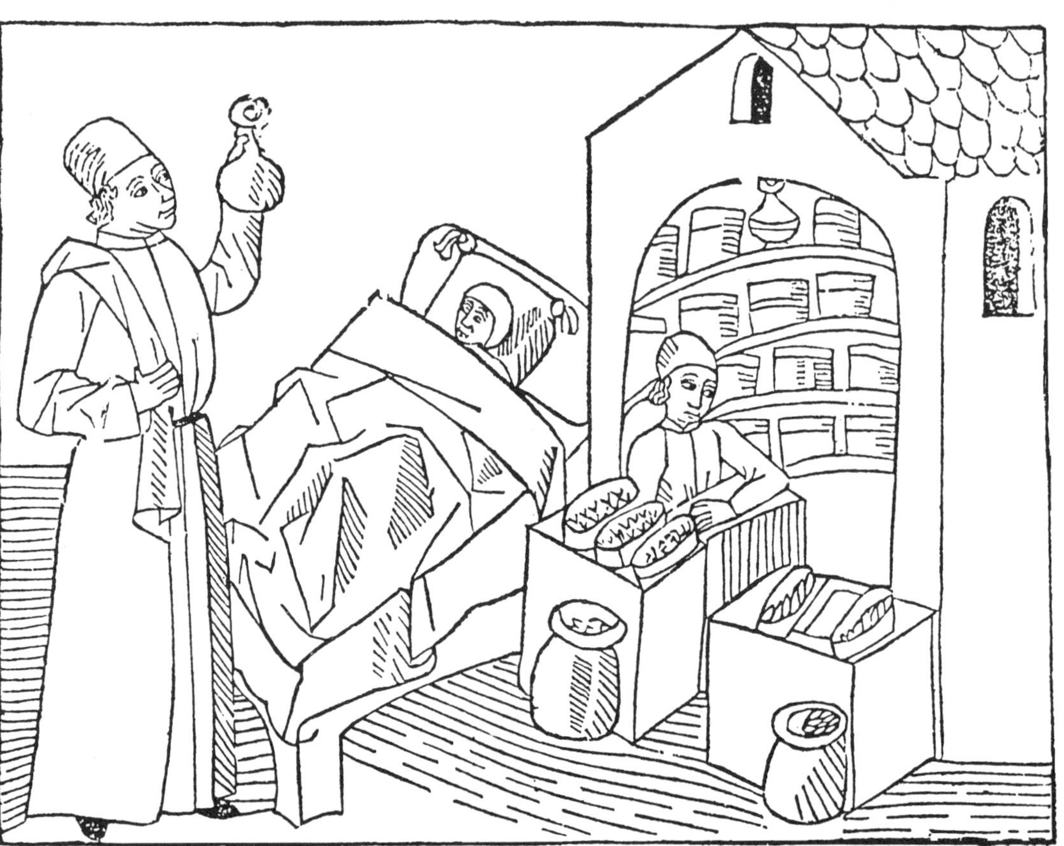

HEALTH VERSUS DISEASE

1. Plato: Body and Mind in Health and Disease

Today we talk about and study agents of disease and observed alterations in structure and function of tissues and organs. There are some precise cures available for certain precise diagnoses (for example, certain bacterial infections), but for many chronic diseases we remain far from a fundamental understanding of their processes. Atherosclerosis, chronic arthritis, mental disease, and solid malignant neoplasms come readily to mind. Today we comprehend the scientific basis for many aspects of these disorders and are able to treat them to some extent but are still struggling to comprehend the underlying causes and the means of preventing them. In some ways the helplessness before human maladies of the ancient Greeks in Plato's era still vexes us today. Plato, writing in *Charmides* and *The Republic,* helps set the context for disease, reminds us to treat the whole patient.

I dare say that you have heard eminent physicians say to a patient who comes to them with bad eyes that they cannot cure his eyes by themselves, but that if his eyes are to be cured, his head must be treated; and then again they say that to think of curing the head alone, and not the rest of the body also, is the height of folly. And arguing in this way they apply their methods to the whole body, and try to treat and heal the whole and the part together.[1]

Even more to the point in what we now call psychosomatic disorders, he advises us as to the importance of the soul.

The Greek physicians are quite right as far as they go; but . . . you ought not to attempt to cure the eyes without the head, or the head without the body, so neither ought you to attempt to cure the body without the soul; and this . . . is the reason why the cure of many diseases is unknown to the physicians of Hellas, because they are ignorant of the whole, which ought to be studied also; for the part can never be well unless the whole is well.[2]

In the political treatise *The Republic*, Plato comments further on the importance of the mind-body relationship.

My own belief is—not that the good body by any bodily excellence improves the soul, but, on the contrary, that the good soul, by her own excellence, improves the body as far as this may be possible.[3]

Even in ancient Greece, patients contributed to their own dysfunction. Excess in diet and drink then and now make medicine more difficult.

Where temperance is, there health is speedily imparted, not only to the head, but to the whole body.[4]

We now know for many good biochemical and physiological reasons that moderation in diet and exercise are important in health maintenance. Plato tells us that as a certain spiritual calmness results from simple musical stimuli so does exercise promote health.

. . . simplicity in music . . . the parent of temperance in the soul; and simplicity in gymnastic of health in the body.[5]

Hypochondriasis is not a new phenomenon. It seems in Plato's Athens that many a self-indulgent patient demanded treatment, and the medical practitioners obliged.

To require the help of medicine, not when a wound has to be cured, or on occasion of an epidemic, but just because, by indolence and a habit of life such as we have been describing, men fill themselves with waters and winds, as if their bodies were a marsh, compelling the ingenious sons of Asclepius to find more names for diseases, such as flatulence and catarrh; is not this, too, a disgrace?[6]

Different schools of medical practice—specialists versus generalists, surgeons versus internists—approach patient management in different ways. Patients then and now also deal with their doctors in different ways.

When a carpenter is ill he asks the physician for a rough and ready cure; an emetic or a purge or a cautery or the knife. . . . If someone prescribes for him a course of dietetics . . . he replies that he has no time to be ill . . . and therefore bidding good-bye to this sort of physician, he resumes his ordinary habits, and either gets well and lives and does his business, or, if his constitution fails, he dies and has no more trouble.[7]

As we face in medicine today the difficult issues of possible rationing of care and of considering measures of quality as well as length of life, Plato gives us a political analogy that touches on the issues involved:

Therefore our politic Asclepius may be supposed to have exhibited the power of his art only to persons who, being

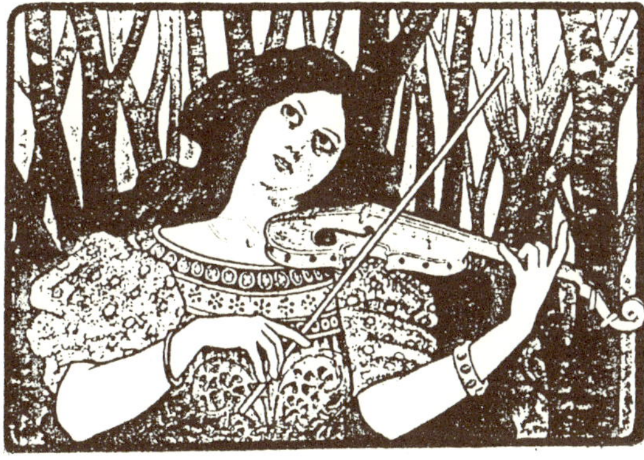

Simple music tempers both soul and body.

generally of healthy constitution and habits of life had a definite ailment; such as these he cured by purges and operations, and bade them live as usual, herein consulting the interests of the State; but bodies which disease had penetrated through and through he would not have attempted to cure by gradual processes of evacuation and infusion: he did not want to lengthen out good-for-nothing lives, or to have weak fathers begetting weaker sons—if a man was not able to live in the ordinary way he had no business to cure him; for such a cure would have been of no use either to himself, or to the State.[8]

Herodicus [a member of the guild of Asclepius] by a combination of training and doctoring found out a way of torturing first and chiefly himself, and secondly the rest of the world . . . by the invention of lingering death; for he had a mortal disease which he perpetually tended, and as recovery was out of the question, he passed his entire life as a valetudinarian; he could do nothing but attend upon himself, and he was in constant torment whenever he departed in anything from his usual regimen, and so dying hard, by the help of science he struggled on to old age.[9]

An especially acute aspect of this problem is present when doctors today confront the issue of saving life versus prolonging the process of dying in the intensive care unit. Managing dying patients is and has always been stressful for both doctor and patient. Plato gives us another example showing how a patient's perception of his disease can complicate life; even when the disease is not so severe as believed, the reaction to it by the patient can be all-consuming.

In contrast to this case, in which the effect of medical therapy seems questionable, it is remarkable that a doctor's efforts to preserve and extend life, when truly and immediately threatened by severe disease, often succeed, occasionally miraculously, against all odds; but in some cases the physician's efforts paradoxically may add to the total burden for the patient and the family in the difficult transition from life to death, especially when the patient is beyond all consciousness or hope. In some of these instances, the doctor is

torn between intervening or not; after all, hope-
less patients have recovered and hopeful patients
have lived for long periods of time, never recov-
ering. For the physician treating such patients,
the choices can be tormenting. The consequences of medical intervention, ordinary or extraordinary, present the physician repeatedly with
difficult choices and require hard decisions where
there are no easy answers.

2. Hippocrates: Profession or Trade Guild?

Hippocrates was a historical figure, but many of the writings attributed to him are generally held to represent rather a school of thought or the collected works of many contributors. Some see the writings as early statements of a still valid philosophical approach to medicine that takes the whole patient into consideration and warns the physician not to harm the patient. Others view the Hippocratic oath (see frontispiece) more cynically—merely as the expression of a way of preserving the basis for a restrictive money-making guild. In spite of these disparate points of view about the oath, certain elements expressed there and elsewhere in the Hippocratic works are to this day valued in modern medical practice. Clearly manifest in this body of work are attitudinal approaches to patient care that doctors still are striving to maximize.

Such attributes as thoroughness, reliability, analytical ability, and efficiency are still inculcated as desirable by medical professors into their students. Then, as now, there was an attempt to define diseases as natural processes with logical sequences. The physician ought to be able to observe, classify, and predict the outcome of the various human diseases. These age-old elements are part of our present sequence: history and physical examination, diagnosis, prognosis. Today, of course, we go much beyond the four elements of Empedocles:

For if hot, or cold, or moist, or dry, be
that which proves injurious to man, and if
the person who would treat him properly
must apply cold to the hot, hot to the cold,
moist to the dry, and dry to the moist. . . .[10]

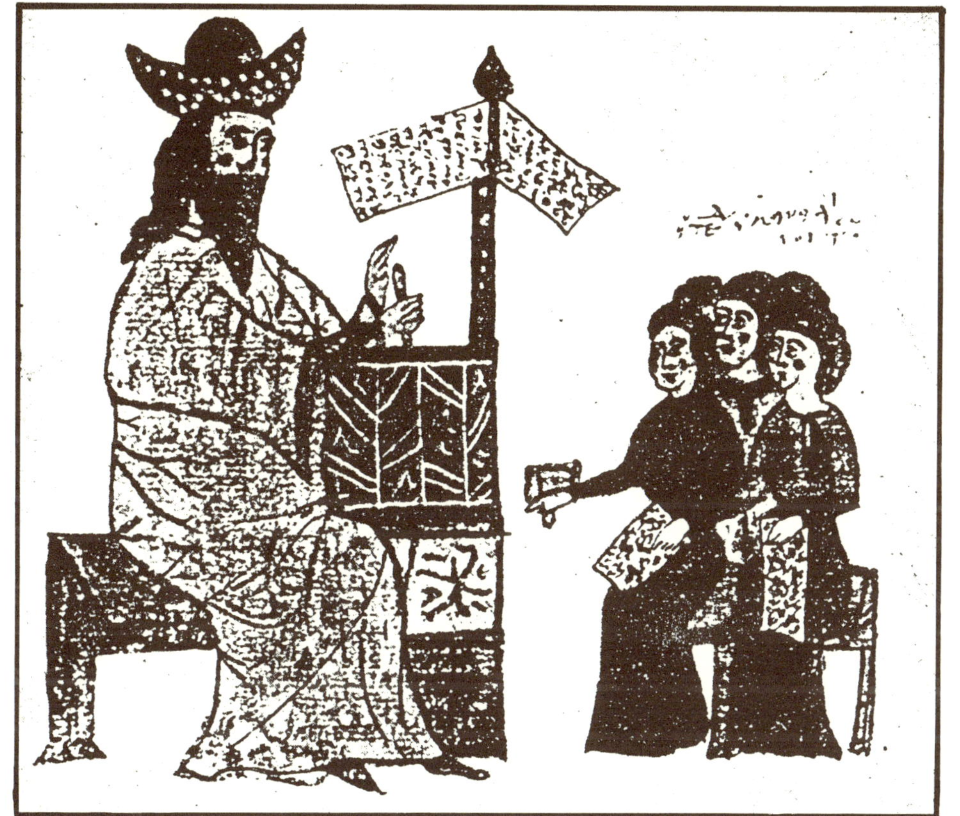

*The great Hippocrates
teaching his students.*

Some of these tenets are still adhered to. Cold is, to this day, applied to muscle and joint sprains right after injury to reduce swelling and inflammation. In fevers, antipyretic medications such as aspirin and acetaminophen are given to reduce fever. In some instances, extraordinary means are used to slow down metabolic processes, for example, physically cooling the circulating extracorporeal blood during some types of cardiac surgery. Cautious warming is indicated for hypothermia. Dry bandages are frequently used to absorb exudate leaking from surgical wounds, and some dry-skin conditions are treated with wet or moist dressings.

The Hippocratic school emphasized the importance of the individual's overall constitution. Each patient's special circumstance is still a cardinal element in the training of student doctors to evaluate and treat patients:

> They did not suppose that the dry or the moist, the hot or the cold, or any of these are either injurious to man, or that man stands in need of them, but whatever in each was strong, and more than a match for a man's constitution, whatever he could not manage, that they held to be hurtful, and sought to remove.[11]

Special treatments were to be designed for each particular patient. This approach still applies and is a major part of what we call the art of medicine by professional judgment, as opposed to medicine by cookbook, *Reader's Digest,* or rote list-checking.

Current principles of disease are much more complex than the then popular theory of humors:

> Thus, when there is an overflow of the bitter principle, which we call yellow bile, what anxiety, burning heat, and loss of strength prevail! But if relieved from it, either by being purged spontaneously, or by means of a medicine seasonably administered, the patient is decidedly relieved of the pains and heat.[12]

The word "bilious," although no longer used in the above sense medically, still has the same connotation in general speech.

In *On Regimen in Acute Diseases,* we learn that diet is most important, as we now still believe; but the ancients thought that the substance of the diet was less important in causing disease than an abrupt change. We now know that sudden changes can in and of themselves be stressful.

One may derive information from the regimen of persons in good health what things are proper; for if it appear that there is a great difference whether the diet be so and so, in other respects, but more especially in the changes, how can it be otherwise in diseases, and more especially in the most acute? But it is well ascertained that even a faulty diet of food and drink, steadily persevered in, is safer in the main as regards health than if one suddenly change it to another.[13]

3. Aristotle: Biological Perspective on Man

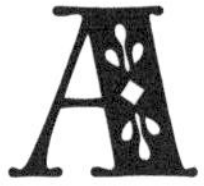ristotle's influence has been enormous through the ages and to this day remains pervasive. He pointed out that blood was important and that observations on animals can be applied to understanding human disease:

> Animals that are in good condition, either from natural causes or from their health having been attended to, have the blood neither too abundant—as creatures just after drinking have the liquid inside them in abundance—nor again very scanty, as is the case with animals when exceedingly fat.[14]

Body composition seems to have been thought important in health even in ancient Athens. Now, of course, we know about water distribution in various tissues, the effects of adiposity on metabolic and endocrine function, and even fat cell hyperplasia's role in obesity. What we would now call a neuroendocrine dysfunction or emotional eating disorder may well have been what Aristotle was talking about when he related the vigor of the organism to its form or constitution:

> Both men and women are liable to constitutional change, growing healthier or more sickly, or altering in the way of leanness, stoutness, and vigour.[15]

Aristotle reminds us of the importance of proportionality and hints at what we now call feedback loops or servomechanisms:

> Wherever the action of any part is in excess, nature so contrives as to set by it another part with an excess of contrary action, so that the excesses of the two may counterbalance each other.[16]

His theory of the ice cold versus red hot brain does not coincide with what we now know about neurophysiology, but the importance he attaches to blood surfaced centuries later in Harvey's works:

> For if the brain be either too fluid or too solid, it will not perform its office, but in the one case will freeze the blood, and in the other will not cool it at all; and thus will cause disease, madness, and death. For the cardiac heat and the center of life is most delicate in its sympathies, and is immediately sensitive to the slightest change or affection of the blood on the outer surface of the brain.[17]

In *Parts of Animals*, Aristotle elaborates on the humoral theory, more fully expounded by Galen, and implies that physicians ought to assay body fluids as to sweetness and bitterness—assays that we do now with instruments to measure blood glucose and pH rather than with our tongues. Here Aristotle postulates a relationship between blood and bile:

> When animals are formed of blood less pure in composition, the bile serves for the excretion of its impure residue. For the very meaning of excrement is that it is the opposite of nutriment, and of bitter that it is the opposite of sweet; and healthy blood is sweet. So that it is evident that the bile, which is bitter, cannot have any useful end, but must simply be a purifying excretion.[18]

The insight shown here into the excretory function of bile is extraordinary!

We no longer believe that the liver in and of itself determines the length of life; yet, on the other hand, high-density and low-density lipoproteins are produced in that organ, and we now know there is a relation between hepatic lipoprotein metabolism and life-ending cardiovascular disease. Here is what Aristotle has to say about the liver and length of life:

> Seeing, indeed, that the liver is not only useful, but a necessary and vital part in all animals that have blood, it is but reasonable that on its character should depend the length or the shortness of life.[19]

Aristotle reminds us of how important good health is to us and our patients. Patients tend to focus more on loss of function, on diminished capacity for activities of daily living or diminished enjoyment of life—in all its varieties—as a consequence of loss of good health. Doctors tend to focus more on diseases or specific organ dysfunction and the maintenance of specific biological functions to such an extent that it sometimes impedes their understanding of just what it is that troubles sick people. Aristotle points out in *Rhetoric* that

> The excellence of the body is health; that
> is, a condition which allows us, while
> keeping free from disease, to have the use
> of our bodies.[20]

Good health allows full enjoyment of life; doctors may give so much attention to specific biological or biochemical defects that they must be reminded on occasion, as in this instance by Aristotle, to consider the overall quality of a patient's life along with the serum electrolyte concentrations and the creatinine clearance.

Some of our contemporary concerns about health maintenance concentrate on various ill effects of self-chosen habits or activities. Aristotle pointed out an attitude expressed by twentieth-century men and women fearful of the consequences of smoking, drinking, overeating, and sexually transmitted diseases:

> Many people are "healthy" . . . and these
> no one can congratulate on their "health,"
> for they have to abstain from everything or
> nearly everything that men do.[21]

Health and happiness go hand in hand as conventional wisdom to this day tells us. But in medicine, then as now, relationships are not always simple:

> Happiness in old age is the coming of old
> age slowly and painlessly. . . . It arises
> both from the excellences of the body and
> from good luck. If a man is not free from
> disease, or if he is not strong, he will not
> be free from suffering; nor can he continue
> to live a long and painless life unless he
> has good luck.[22] [On the other hand]
> [t]here is, indeed a capacity for long life
> that is quite independent of health or
> strength; for many people live long who
> lack the excellences of the body.[23]

In medicine, then and now, much to our chagrin as prognosticators, the exception proves the rule.

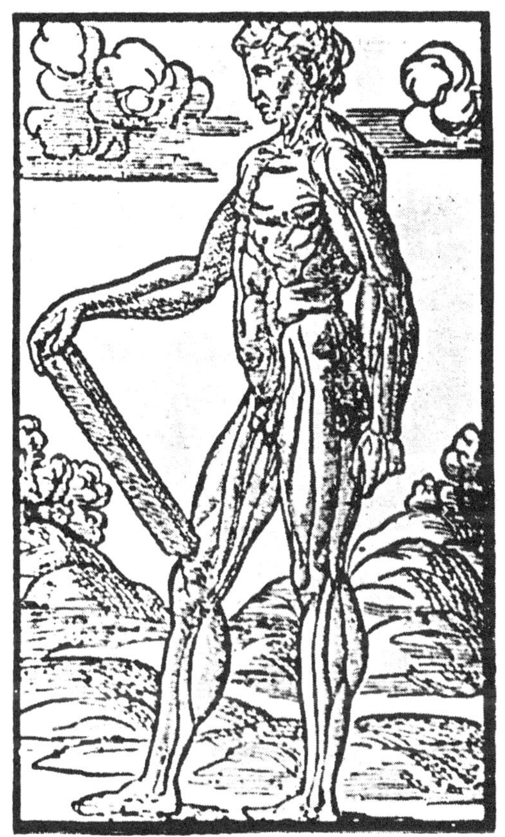 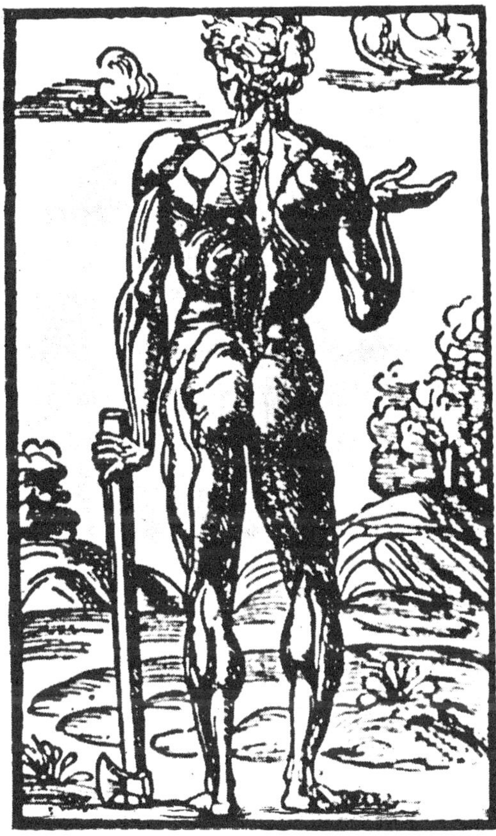

A well-toned musculature allows full enjoyment of life.

♦ 15 ♦

4. Galen: The Physician, a Philosopher?

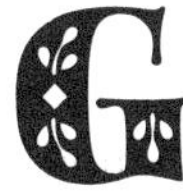Galen dominated medicine in his dogmatic way for centuries, and his theories are now soundly rejected; but some of his recorded observations still merit study and consideration. Implicit in his works is a vivid perception of the healing power of nature, a theme that recurs again and again in all recorded annals of medicine.

The Aristotelian role of disharmony or imbalance was still important to Galen; he was, after all, a Greek physician of the Alexandrian school although he practiced in the Roman Empire. He tells us about disproportion and disease:

> But, indeed, if disproportion of heat belongs to the primary diseases, it cannot but be that a proportionate blending [eucrasia] of the qualities produces the normal activity. For a disproportionate blend [dyscrasia] can only become a cause of the primary diseases through derangement of the eucrasia. That is to say, it is because the [normal] activities arise from the eucrasia that the primary impairments of these activities necessarily arise from its derangement.[24]

Galen tells us a great deal about the humoral theory, explaining first of all that the four humors—blood, yellow bile, black bile, and phlegm or mucus—are generated in the body.[25] When functions are normal, blood (the warm and moist humor) predominates and there is eucrasia[26] or proportionate blending of temperature; the body is at normal temperature. When there is too much heat, yellow bile (the warm and dry humor) predominates as is often the case in warm periods of life, in warm countries, at warm seasons of the year, and in people of warm temperaments. Similarly, yellow bile is excessive in warm occupations, ways of life, and diseases.[27] Phlegm (the cold and moist humor) is associated with diseases following wet, chilling experiences (for example, colds and pneumonia), whereas black bile (the cold and dry humor) is associated with mental depression and aging. In doing this explaining, he repeats the then centuries old dicta of the Hippocratic school.

> Bodies act upon and are acted upon by each other in virtue of the Warm, Cold, Moist, and Dry. And if one is speaking of any activity, whether it be exercised by vein, liver, arteries, heart, alimentary canal, or any part, one will be inevitably compelled to acknowledge that this activity depends upon the way in which the four qualities are blended.[28]

Some of Galen's commentary to Roman medical practitioners in the second century A.D. is still valid and forms the basis of part of the modern medical school curriculum:

For how are you going to be successful in treatment if you do not understand the real essence of each disease?[29] . . . It is in our power to alter and transmute morbid states of the body—in fact, to give them a turn for the better. But if we did not know in what respect they were morbid or in what way they diverged from the normal, how should we be able to ameliorate them?[30]

We still teach medical students that a thorough understanding of disease is a fundament for good medical practice. Though from a vastly different perspective, we still emphasize correlates of altered form and function:

> The actual disease is that condition of the body which, not accidentally, but primarily and of itself, impairs the normal function.[31]

Galen first tells us quite directly:

> There have arisen . . . two sects in medicine and philosophy . . . who realize the logical sequence of their hypotheses, and stand by them . . . . The one class

supposes that all substance which is subject
to genesis and destruction is at once
continuous and susceptible of alteration.
The other school assumes substance to be
unchangeable, unalterable, and subdivided
into fine particles, which are separated
from one another by empty spaces.[32]

Then he tells us to think for ourselves and make
up our minds as to what we believe and be definite about it:

Those who cannot understand even this,
but who simply talk any nonsense that
comes to their tongues, and who do not
remain definitely attached either to one
sect or the other—such people are not
even worth mentioning.[33]

Affirming what you believe, thinking on your
feet, deciding for yourself—these are traits still
treasured in medical schools, encouraged in students.

Words we still use in everyday language are
based upon Galenic temperamental classifications. Consider:

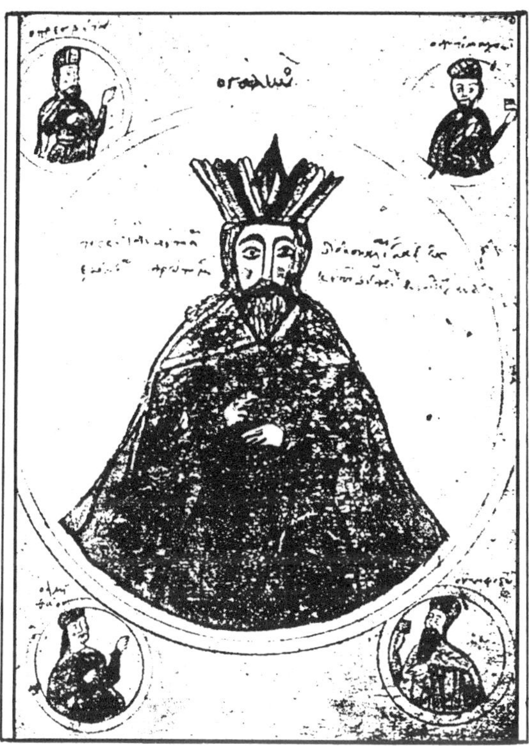

*Galen . . . as Philosopher
King?*

Sanguine—
Blood is virtually warm and moist
humor.[34]

We have a sanguine outlook when things are in
balance and going well. We are cheerful and con-
fident with a ruddy complexion. Blood and its
redness predominate.

Bilious—
Yellow bile is warm and dry (even though
for the most part it appears moist).[!][35]

When it is excessive we are bilious, that is,
cranky, irritable, or peevish, as can well be the
case when there is an intestinal obstruction and
bile backs up into the stomach, coloring its contents yellow.

Phlegmatic—
Phlegm, the over-roasted humor, is cold
and moist. . . . Mucus is the . . . humor
which collects mostly in old people and in
those who have been chilled in some way,
and not even a lunatic could say that this
was anything else than cold and moist.[36]

Persons with severe collections of airway mucus
are apt to be sluggish or apathetic, perhaps from
lack of oxygen.

Melancholic—
Cold and dry . . . black bile is such a
humour. . . . [It] tends to be in excess
mainly in the fall of the year and . . .
mainly after the prime of life.[37]

Gloomy melancholy or clinical depression occurs
more often in midlife or older patients.

The humoral theory that originated in ancient
Greece endured for centuries, even until the time
of William Harvey, when new perspectives on
the differences between health and disease, based
on experimentation and anatomical studies, were
established.

5. Harvey: Observations Are Important

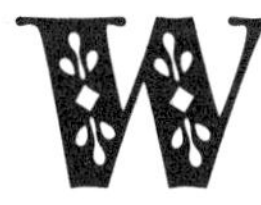illiam Harvey based his conclusions on the circulation of blood upon anatomical observations and experimental work; his writings reflect the heritage of the humoral theory but encourage physicians to take a look for themselves. Harvey emphasized the importance of the heart, blood, and circulatory system in disease but also appreciated the role of emotion in disease:

> Hence it is that if the heart be unaffected,
> life and health may be restored to almost
> all the other parts of the body; but the
> heart being chilled or smitten with a
> serious disease, it seems matter of necessity
> that the whole animal fabric should suffer
> and fall into decay.[38]

Many practitioners of modern psychosomatic medicine would agree with Harvey in the following, wherein he points out the strong effect of emotion in human disease:

> Grief and love, and envy and anxiety, and
> all affections of the mind of a similar kind
> are accompanied with emaciation and
> decay, or with cacochemy and crudity,
> which engender all manner of diseases and
> consume the body of man. For every
> affection of the mind that is attended with
> either pain or pleasure, hope or fear, is the
> cause of an agitation whose influence
> extends to the heart, and there induces
> change from the natural constitution, in
> the temperature, the pulse and the rest.[39]

In *Animal Generation*, he reiterates the preeminent role he attaches to the humor blood in life:

The blood acts, then, with forces superior to the forces of the elements. . . . It is possessed by a soul which is not only vegetative, but sensitive and motive also; it penetrates everywhere and is ubiquitous; abstracted, the soul or the life too is gone, so that the blood does not seem to differ in any respect from the soul of the life itself (anima); at all events, it is to be regarded as the substance whose act is the soul or the life.[40]

His judgment seems to us distorted by an exclusive consideration of the performance of the circulatory system. On the other hand, even today we use blood as our primary source of raw material for diagnostic laboratory testing and recognize the extreme importance of maintaining adequate circulation in sick patients. Also, we now realize the importance of then unrecognized but vital refinements of the circulatory system such as those manifest in the hepatic and hypothalamic-pituitary portal systems. Harvey writes:

The blood, therefore, even as the soul, is to be regarded as the cause and author of youth and old age, of sleep and waking, and also of respiration; all the more and especially as the first instrument in natural things contains the internal moving cause within itself. It therefore comes to the same thing, whether we say that the soul and the blood, or the blood with the soul, or the soul with the blood, performs all the acts in the animal organism.[41]

Thomas Aquinas agrees with Harvey:

One sickness is graver than another. For just as the good of health consists in a certain balance of the humors in keeping with an animal's nature, so the good of virtue consists in a certain proportion of the human act in accord with the rule of reason. Now it is evident that the higher the principle whose disorder causes the disorder in the humors, the graver is the sickness; thus a sickness which comes on the human body from the heart, which is the principle of life, or from some neighboring part, is more dangerous.[42]

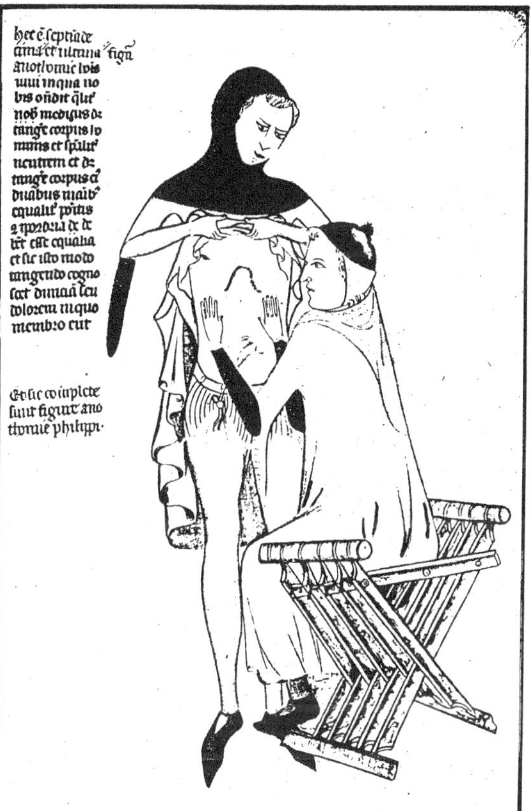

hic é septiade
aim et ultima figu
anothomie lvis
uui inqua no
bis oñdit qur
nob medcius de
tangit corpus lo
nums et spuit
licutrem et de
tangit corpus ca
duabus maib
cqualit portis
q mozora de te
irt est cqualia
et sic isto modo
ungtudo cogno
scat dimaañ seu
volorem niquo
membro cut

Et sic complete
sunt figure ano
thomie philippi

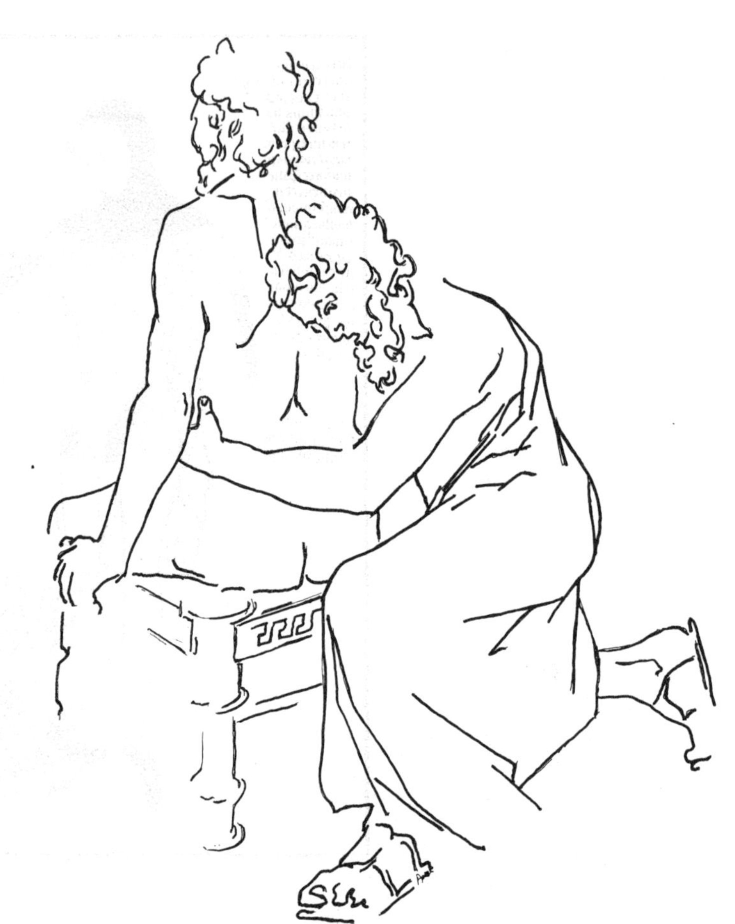

THE NATURE OF DISEASE

6. Plato and Hobbes: Analogies between the Body and the State

Plato, in *The Republic,* reminds us that diseases are principally a manifestation of disorder. Just as health is strong and the natural order of the body, so is virtue of the soul; on the other hand, vice and diseases are defects, one of the soul the other of the body:

> And the creation of health is the institution of a natural order and government of one by another in the parts of the body; and the creation of disease is the production of a state of things at variance with this natural order. . . . Then virtue is the health and beauty and well-being of the soul, and vice the disease and weakness and deformity of the same.[43]

He further likens the body of the person to the governmental state:

> As in a body which is diseased the addition of a touch from without may bring on illness, and sometimes even when there is no external provocation a commotion may arise within—in the same way wherever there is weakness in the State there is also likely to be illness, of which the occasions may be very slight, the one party introducing from without their oligarchical, the other their democratical allies, and then the State falls sick, and is at war with herself and may be at times distracted even when there is no external cause.[44]

When external causes are not evident, then an internal imbalance is most likely at work.

In *Timaeus,* in another context, he attributes disease to what we would probably term a disordered biochemical mechanism:

Diseases . . . owe their severity to the fact that the generation of these substances [earth, fire, air, water] proceeds in a wrong order; they are then destroyed.[45]

We still teach that in many circumstances the integrity of the underlying support or framework of an organ is critical to regeneration of function. Plato tells us:

When the several parts of the flesh are separated by disease, if the foundation remains, the power of the disorder is only half as great, and there is still a prospect of an easy recovery; but when that which binds the flesh to the bones is diseased . . . [it] makes the . . . disorders still greater.[46]

It is worse still when the foundation structure itself decays or falls apart. In osteomyelitis or severe bone infection just that may happen. He gives us an example that contains some accuracies about what can happen to bone in osteomyelitis but for reasons quite different from what we understand them to be in the twentieth century.

Still worse are the prior disorders; as when the bone itself, by reason of the density of the flesh, does not obtain sufficient air, but becomes mouldy and hot and gangrened and receives no nutriment, and the natural process is inverted, and the bone crumbling passes into the food, and the food into the flesh, and the flesh again falling into the blood makes all maladies that may occur more virulent.[47]

Sepsis or bacterial infection of the blood is a serious complication which may lead to death. In it the circulating blood transports bacteria throughout the body, permeating into all its parts. It can arise from osteomyelitis, and the severity of some types of this disease was recognized by Plato. He tells us that when the very center of the bone or foundation structure is involved, the prognosis is worse still.

The worst case of all is when the marrow is diseased, either from excess or defect; and this is the cause of the very greatest and most fatal disorders, in which the whole course of the body is reversed.[48]

Human bodies then become corrupt and decay, just as states do when there is damage to the foundation structures, especially when the seat of the lesion is in the core or center of the support.

In *Symposium,* Plato relates the difference between health and disease and the desirability of one over the other:

> There are in the human body these two
> kinds of love . . . the desire of the
> healthy is one, and the desire of the
> diseased is another.[49]

What doctors do is to discourage the desire or elements of disease:

> In the body the good and healthy elements
> are to be indulged, and the bad elements
> and the elements of disease are not to be
> indulged, but discouraged. And this is
> what the physician has to do, and in this
> the art of medicine consists: for medicine
> may be regarded generally as the
> knowledge of the loves and desires of the
> body, and how to satisfy them or not; and

> the best physician is he who is able to
> separate fair love from foul, or to convert
> one into the other; and he who knows
> how to eradicate and how to implant love,
> whichever is required, and can reconcile
> the most hostile elements in the
> constitution and make them loving friends,
> is a skilful practitioner. . . . The most
> hostile are the most opposite, such as hot
> and cold, bitter and sweet, moist and dry,
> and the like.[50]

Knowledge of human nature, its seems, is crucial to the practice of medicine. Not too many modern physicians would quarrel with this assertion.

Centuries later, in Hobbes' *Leviathan,* we again encounter analogies between governments and civil disorder and the human body and disease. In a comparison to the circumstance in which more than one entity claims sovereignty in a commonwealth, he tells us about seizure disorders:

> And this is a disease which not unfitly may
> be compared to the epilepsy, or falling
> sickness . . . in the body natural. For as
> in this disease there is an unnatural spirit

or wind in the head that obstructeth the roots of the nerves and, moving them violently, taketh away the motion which naturally they should have from the power of the soul in the brain; and thereby causeth violent and irregular motions, which men call convulsions.[51]

Raising money for war evokes a response similar to chills and fever.

> . . . ague; wherein, the fleshy parts being congealed, or by venomous matter obstructed, the veins which by their natural course empty themselves into the heart, are not (as they ought to be) supplied from the arteries whereby there succeedeth at first a cold contraction and trembling of the limbs; and afterwards a hot and strong endeavor of the heart to force a passage for the blood; and before it can do that, contenteth itself with the small refreshments of such things as cool for a time, till, if nature be strong enough, it break at last the contumacy of the parts obstructed, and dissipateth the venom into sweat; or, if nature be too weak, the patient dieth.[52]

Other observations from this political scientist and philosopher are more directly medical and not inaccurate:

> Blood in a pleurisy, getting into the membrane of the breast, breedeth there an inflammation, accompanied with a fever and painful stitches.[53]

Further comments are certainly at odds with what we now know about genetics but reflect a familiar biblical theme; the sins of the father shall be visited on their sons:

> . . . defectous procreation . . . as the bodies of children gotten by diseased parents are subject either to untimely death, or to purge the ill quality derived from their vicious conception, by breaking out in biles and scabs.[54]

7. Aristotle: General Observations on Health and Disease

Aristotle's categorical observations on health and disease may help explain medicine's traditional focus on disease rather than wellness. Doctors tend to look for particular diseases or diagnoses that they can deal with or treat. While certainly desirable, the state of health or wellness has not been the traditional central arena of medical concern:

> Health in general is the contrary of
> disease, whereas a particular disease, being
> a species of disease, e.g., fever and
> ophthalmia and any other particular
> disease, has no contrary.[55]

Aging, now developing into the principal concern of the developing medical specialty of gerontology, has long stimulated expressions of the similarities between it and disease or comment on the propensity for old age to be associated with disease:

> As the body declines in vigour we tend to
> cold at every time of life, and especially in
> old age, this age being cold and dry. We
> must remember that the nutriment coming
> to each part of the body is concocted by
> the heat appropriate to the part; if the heat
> is inadequate the part loses its efficiency,
> and destruction or disease results.[56]

Peripheral circulatory disorders were then, as now, more common in the elderly:

> In sickness the whole body is deficient in
> natural heat.[57]

Sometimes older patients may die for no clearly discernible reason. We look hard for one, and medical examiners do not accept old age as an adequate cause of death; but perhaps Aristotle had an insight that we have since lost. In our zeal we may have lost sight of the observation that

> We may rightly call disease an acquired
> old age, old age a natural disease; at any
> rate, some diseases produce the same
> effects as old age.[58]

The long prevalent miasmic theory of disease has ancient roots and fanciful explanations for natural phenomena:

> As there is a decay of water, of earth, and
> all such material bodies, so there is also of
> the earthy vapour, for instance what is
> called mould (for mould is a decay of
> earthy vapour). . . . All earthy vapour
> [is] equivalent to thick air.[59]

Vapors were for centuries associated with illness and disease. Even today, one can hear the expression "an attack of the vapors," usually referring to an ill-understood medical incapacitation.

Aristotle reminds us of the bases for differences of opinion about matters of health in the lay population. Different persons, families, or cultures vary as to their beliefs about what is "good for you." Physicians must deal with particular cases, with particular patients, just as navigators must deal with particular ships, in particular waters, under particular weather conditions.

> Questions of what is good for us have no
> fixity, any more than matters of
> health. . . . Particular cases . . . do not
> fall under any art or precept but the agents
> themselves must in each case consider
> what is appropriate to the occasion, as
> happens also in the art of medicine or of
> navigation.[60]

Moderation is recommended by medical practitioners to their patients. Aristotle states:

> It is the nature of such things [as health]
> to be destroyed by defect and excess. . . .
> Drink or food which is above or below a
> certain amount destroys the health, while
> that which is proportionate both produces
> and increases and preserves it.[61]

Physician-scientists of our century will not quibble with this assertion. Most will teach it to their students.

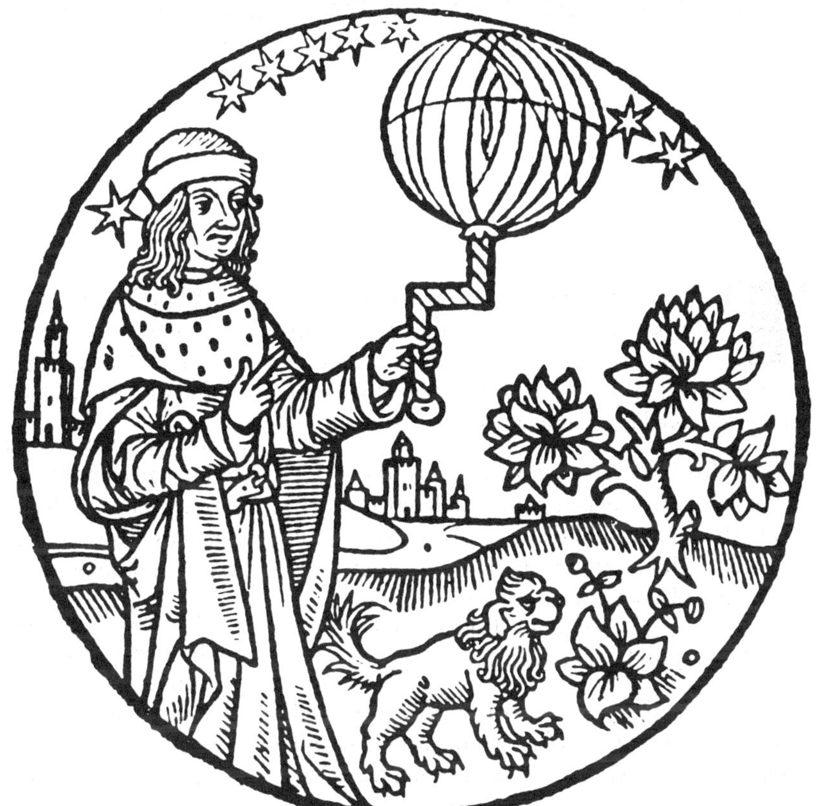

To medieval physicians,
Aristotle's medicine was a
complete, closed sphere.

8. Hippocrates: We Are What We Eat

Traditional Greek medicine emphasized the clinical context of the patient in trying to understand human sickness. As mentioned in earlier chapters, diet has long been considered quite important.

And this I know, moreover, that to the human body it makes a great difference whether the bread be fine or coarse, of wheat with or without the hull, whether mixed with much or little water, strongly wrought or scarcely at all, baked or raw—and a multitude of similar differences.[62]

The early Hippocratic writings constituted quite an exposition of what we today might call human ecology. Medical students then were reminded that

Whoever pays no attention to these things, or, paying attention, does not comprehend them, how can he understand the diseases which befall a man?[63]

The dogma was that natural elements with certain perceptible differences were present in various pairs in balance; when one feature became excessive or noticeable, the consequence was extraordinary:

For there is in man the bitter and the salt, the sweet and the acid, the sour and the insipid, and a multitude of other things having all sorts of powers both as regards quantity and strength. These, when all mixed and mingled up with one another, are not apparent, neither do they hurt a

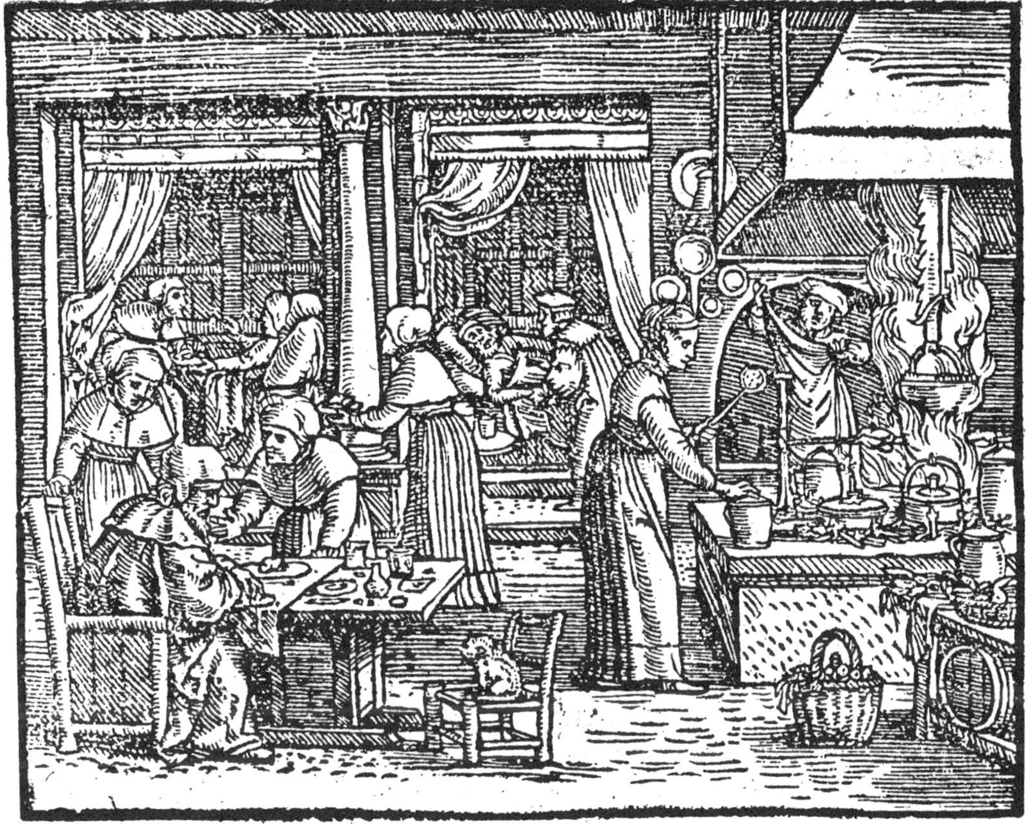

Hippocrates' holistic regimen calls for a varied diet and adequate rest.

man; but when any of them is separate,
and stands by itself, then it becomes
perceptible, and hurts a man.[64]

The nature of the mix of the overall diet as well as the identity of individual constituents was important; just as the powers and tastes of bodily constituents listed above were present in health in moderation and isolated excess in diseases, so dietary constituents in a balanced mixture were healthful. Anything that stood out as well marked or intense was harmful:

All those things which a man eats and
drinks are devoid of any such intense and
well-marked quality, such as bread, cake,
and many other things of a similar nature
which man is accustomed to use for
food. . . . When received into the body
abundantly, there is no disorder nor
dissolution of the powers belonging to the
body; but strength, growth, and
nourishment result from them, and this
for no other reason than because they
are well mixed, have nothing in
them of immoderate character, nor
anything strong, but the whole forms
one simple and not strong
substance.[65]

9. Galen: Hot versus Cold

The ancient Greeks theorized that the four body humors—blood from the heart, yellow bile from the liver, black bile from the spleen, and phlegm from the brain—determined the body's state in health and disease. These humors were associated with the four elements—fire, air, earth, and water—and each in turn corresponded to a pair of the qualities—hot, cold, dry, and moist. Where did the humors come from? They came from the body in response to the amount of heat applied to nutrients.

> In reference to the genesis of the humours . . . when the nutriment becomes altered in the veins by the innate heat, blood is produced when it is in moderation, and the other humours when it is not in proper proportion.[66]

Those foods felt to be hot would increase bile; those cold, phlegm or mucus.

> Those articles of food, which are by nature warmer are more productive of bile, while those which are colder produce . . . phlegm. . . . Of occupations also, localities and seasons, and, above all natures themselves, the colder are more phlegmatic, and the warmer more bilious.[67]

The prime determinants of disease were based on the various combinations of four fundamental characteristics:

> The diseases which are primary and generic are four in number, and differ from each other in warmth, cold, dryness, and moisture.[68]

. . . Every part functions in its own special way because of the manner in which the four qualities are compounded [and it is] absolutely necessary that the function should be either completely destroyed, or at least hampered, by any damage to the qualities and that thus the animal should fall ill, either as a whole or in certain of its parts.[69]

All of what we now know of the complexities of biochemistry and pathophysiology was in Galen's era unknown and unimaginable. In today's terms, the approach then was to lump and classify by a small number of essential traits rather than to split and subclassify based on the minutest of differences, as we now do.

We now use these differences in detail to strive for a precise diagnosis, but we still need to understand how any particular disease disorders a patient's life. In approaches designed to care for the whole patient, many similar but distinct disorders can be and are considered together in treating and following patients. For example, patients with cancer or high blood pressure may have quite different underlying mechanisms of disease, but as groups they have enough problems in common that medicine has developed general strategies to care for them. The problem in this approach is that, paradoxically, it may become the diagnosis, not the individual patient, that is treated. The subcategorizing of patients based on disease could benefit individual patients if the method resulted in the same degree of attention being given to the detailed aspects of the patient as to the detailed aspects of the disease.

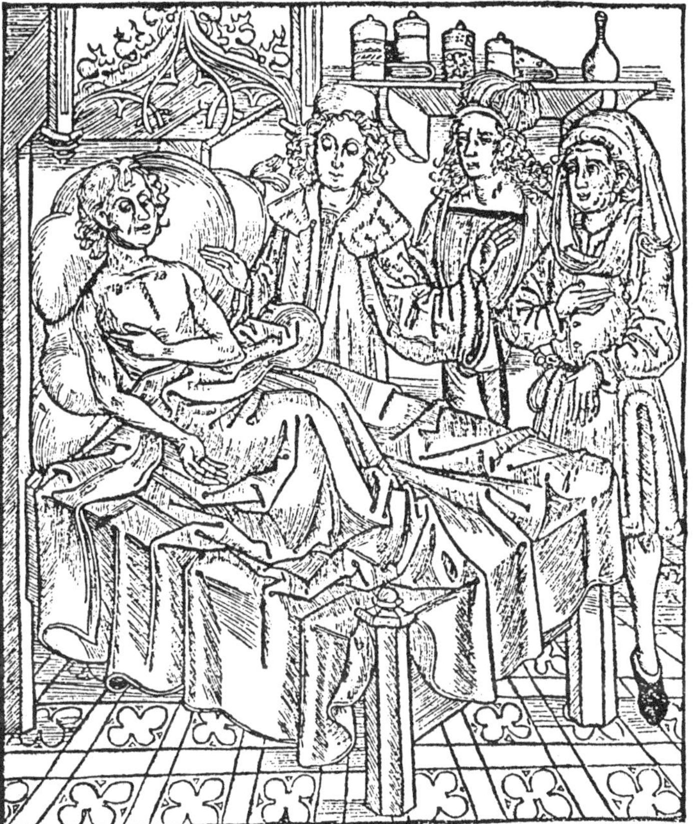

Physicians debate the effects of the humors in a patient.

10. Avicenna: Pneuma—the Vehicle of the Psychic Faculties

In his *Essay on Cardiotherapy* Avicenna, the famous eleventh-century medieval Muslim physician and philosopher, tells us about the then prevalent notion of an airborne vital force:

I say that God the Great made the left one of the ventricles of the heart the source and repository of the pneuma, and created the pneuma as the vehicle of psychic faculties to be carried by it throughout the body. He linked the psychic faculties primarily with the pneuma, and secondarily, through its mediation, made it accessible to all parts of the body. He created the pneuma out of the fine humors and their vaporosity as He created the body out of the gross humors and their earthiness. The relation of the pneuma with the fineness of the humors is similar to the relation of the body with the humors (as a whole). Just as the organs are made out of the humors due to mixing together so as to attain a single temperamental form through which the mixture is enabled to accept the properties (of life) otherwise not attainable by elements, in the same way the substance of the pneuma is made out of the extract of humors due to the mixing of their fair varieties so as to attain a single temperamental form through which the pneuma is enabled to accept psychical faculties otherwise not attainable by elements.[70]

This famous writer wrote a textbook on medicine that reigned as authoritative for several hundred years!

His comments on psychosomatic interactions are interesting:

> If the pneuma that is in the heart is abundant in the material from which it is produced almost continuously, is moderate in temperament and consistency, and bright and luminous, it has a strong capacity for enjoyment. When it is scanty in matter as is the case with the convalescent and persons debilitated by illness and old age, or immoderate in temperament as is the case with the sick, or excessively turbid or thick in consistency as is the case with melancholic and old people, then it does not expand because of its thickness. When it is excessively thin in consistency as with the debilitated men and women, then it does not suffice for expansion. When it is darkened as with the melancholic then it is strongly liable to sadness.[71]

From Avicenna's medieval expressions one can

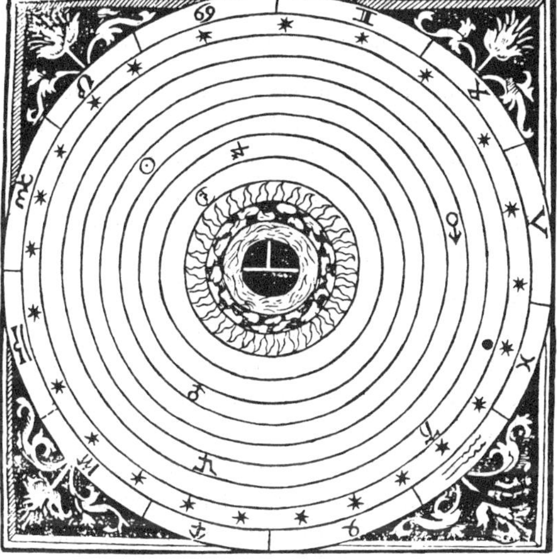

Beyond pneuma, Paracelsus postulates celestial influence on wounds.

realize that some of Harvey's later emphasis on the blood and circulation was not novel:

> Pure and plentiful blood that is moderate in consistency is conducive to joy, since it produces an abundant quantity of pneuma which is pure, brilliant, moderate in consistency and in temperament. Pure blood which is excessive in heat is conducive to anger because of its inflammation and rapid motion. Thin, watery, pure, cold blood tends to produce the weakness of the heart and timidity, because the pneuma which is produced from it becomes sluggish in outward movement and slow to inflame because of its coldness. Thus its capacity for joy and anger is decreased, and it becomes both easily soluble due to its thinness, and difficult to dissolve due to its coldness. Thick, turbid blood, excessive in heat, predisposes to sadness and fixed and insoluble anger. As regards sadness, it comes from the turbid pneuma generated by the blood; as to anger, it is because the blood, by its heat, becomes highly inflammable. As to enduring anger, it is because the blood is thick. When the object which is thick is heated, it does not quickly cool.[72]

We still often use the terms "hot-blooded" and "cold-blooded" to describe different emotional states. A subsequent medieval writer, also living in the Mediterranean-Arabic culture, contributed heavily to the western medical tradition.

11. Maimonides: Gluttony and Sloth—Enemies of Health

In *Regimen Sanitatis*, written in the twelfth century in Arabic, this enduring Jewish philosopher and physician offers insights still considered valid. He repeats many of the thoughts and medical perspectives of the Hippocratic school and of Galen. He asserts the humoral theory and implores the physician to use art, logic, and intuition. He encourages the physician to be what the name "doctor" means—a teacher.

Attention to diet and exercise are still considered important in health maintenance:

[There] are universal precepts of the great physicians . . . . Among these is the statement of Hippocrates that the conservation of health lies in abstaining from repletion and forsaking the disinclination to exertion.[73]

Overeating was and is a human bane; this theme, as we shall see, recurs throughout medical history.

Repletion, that is, eating until the appetite departs and repugnance commences, requires filling the stomach to the utmost of its capacity, and distending it. When any organ becomes distended, its connections are loosened and its vigor is necessarily weakened. The stomach will in no wise digest such a meal adequately. Indolence . . . will occur.[74]

We now look upon hepatic metabolism quite differently; yet, somehow it seems there is some correlation in this description with what our current interpretation of digestion involves:

> When the meal is digested poorly in the stomach, its second digestion in the liver is bound also to be bad, and its third digestion in all the organs will perforce be worst of all. This is the cause of all kinds of diseases in great variety. Galen has said in these words: He who wishes to avoid all illness should take care to avoid indigestion, and should not move about after the meal.[75]

The old Greek idea of moderation has endured:

> To conserve . . . health . . . take in the temperate season an amount [of food] that does not distend the stomach, or burden it and impede the digestion.[76]

Physical exercise consumes calories and activates the body's many systems. It does much more than help control weight!

> Nothing is to be found that can substitute for exercise in any way, because in exercise the natural heat flames up and all the superfluities are expelled, while at rest the flame of the natural heat subsides and superfluities are engendered in the body, even though the food is of the very best quality and is moderate in quantity. And exercise will expel the harm done by most of the bad regimens that most men follow.[77]

Some aspects of what he tells us, in Aristotelian tradition, about lipids would find some support among modern investigators of atherosclerosis:

> Fat is all bad; it surfeits, corrupts the digestion, suppresses the appetite and generates phlegmy humor.[78]

Maimonides reminds us that the physician can help in some cases, but not all. This lesson still provokes debate in the era of modern life-extending medical technology.

> If the vigor of the sick is stronger than the strength of the disease, there is no need for the physician at all; Nature will cure them. But if the disease and the vigor are equal, then the physician is needed to aid the vigor.[79]

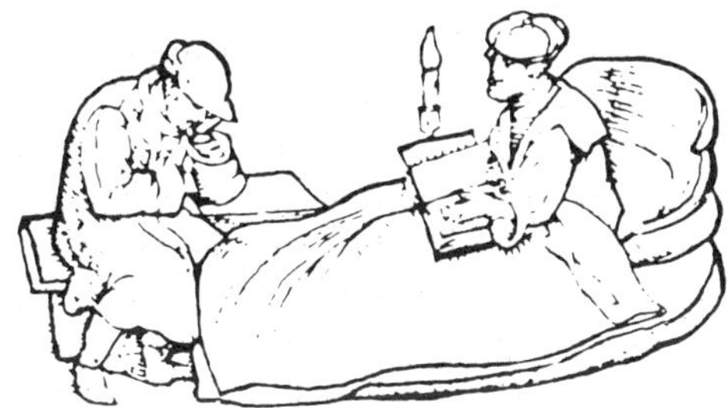

Don't read in bed

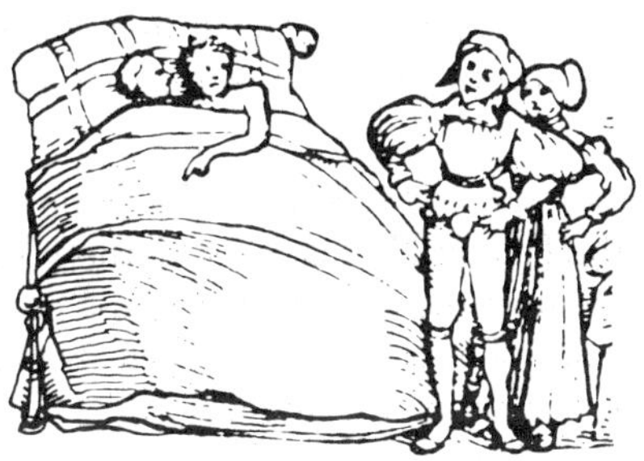

Don't love too much

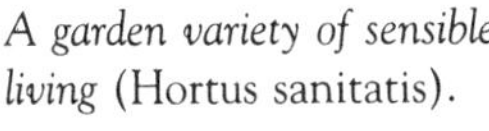

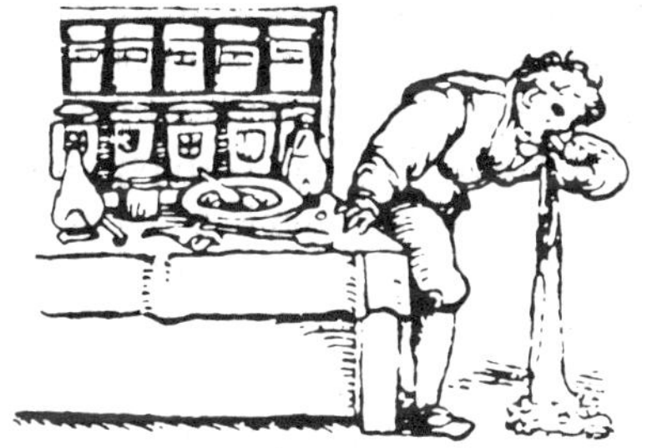

Don't drink too much

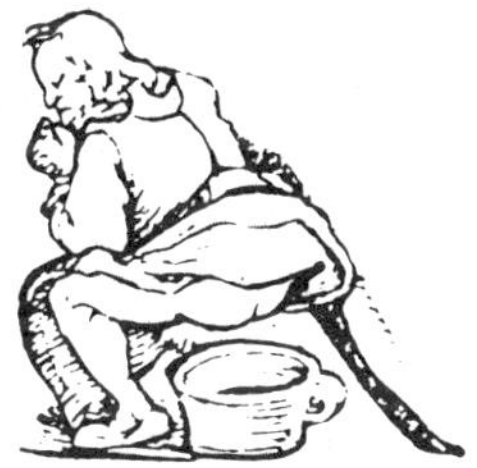

Don't strain too much

Sometimes, he repeats a theme from Plato and Aristotle—the treatment is worse than the disease:

> Aristotle says in his book on Perception and the Perceptible that most of those who die, die from the treatment, because of the ignorance of most physicians about Nature. Physicians mean by Nature, in this connection, that power which governs the bodies of living creatures.[80]

How to choose a personal physician and arrange consultations or second opinions are issues facing us still:

> Kings gather numerous physicians and select from among them those endowed with wisdom, and those of long experience, for perhaps by the coming together of such minds they will be saved from error.[81]

He remains true to his era and repeats the teachings of the ancients and Avicenna on air and the elements:

> First, one ought to attend to the rectification of the air, then to the rectification of the nutrients. This is so because what the physicians call pneumas, are fine vapors found in the body of living creatures; their origin and the main part of their substance are from the air inhaled from without. The vapor of the blood found in the liver and in the veins arising from it is called the Natural Spirit, the vapor of the blood found in the heart and the pulsating vessels is called the Vital Spirit, and the vapor found in the ventricles of the brain and that which is transmitted from it through the cavities of the nerves is called the Psychic Spirit. The source of all these, and most of their substance, is the air inhaled from without, and if this air becomes corrupt, putrid, or turbid, all pneumas undergo alterations and their affairs proceed contrary to what is proper.
>
> The finer the pneuma is, the more it is altered by the changes in the air.[82]

One philosophical observation has some validity, and this written by an eminent physician, sympathetic to physicians!

When all ailments are taken into consideration, the physician can be dispensed with more often than he is needed, even when he is excellent, knows how to assist Nature, and does not perplex her or divert her from her proper pathway.[83]

Modern theorists of neuroimmunology would not agree with the fact nor with the interpretation; yet this description makes interesting reading for the student of medicine:

Always protect the head from the intense cold which causes rheums, and also from the intense heat, because the intense heat melts the coagulated superfluities that are in the brain, and they descend; these are the hot rheums. All the rheums, hot and cold, often pour into the hollows of the lung and fill them all at once, because of the abundance of the descending humor and the weakness of the recipient. The expulsive power is too weak to expel it by cough, and the man suffocates and dies or develops orthopnea. At other times they descend to the hollow of the stomach and cause mucosity of the intestine; this is a disease that is hard to cure. Or at times, they descend to one of the joints, and produce aching of the joints. They can also descend to the substance of the internal organs and their cavities, and produce swelling in these organs, pleurisy, inflammation of the lungs, swelling of the liver, and swelling of the stomach or the rest of the members. Because of this, it is important to beware of rheums.[84]

It should be clear from the above why mothers advise not to sleep in a drafty room with the window open on a cold night!

For a more anatomically oriented view of disease, we move on several centuries—to seventeenth-century Europe.

12. Harvey: Internal Organs Are Altered in Disease!

Dissection of human cadavers is taken for granted by today's medical students, but for centuries it was outlawed. Harvey was one of the first to point out the value of anatomic dissection and especially postmortem examinations:

Not with the purpose . . . of indicating the seats of diseases from the bodies of healthy subjects, and discussing the several diseases that make their appearance there, according to the views which others have entertained of them; but that I may relate from the many dissections I have made of the bodies of persons diseased, worn out by serious and strange affections, how and in what way the internal organs were changed in their situation, size, structure, figure, consistency, and other sensible qualities, from their natural forms and appearances, such as they are usually described by anatomists; and in what various and remarkable ways they were affected. . . .

For even as the dissection of healthy and well-constituted bodies contributes essentially to the advancement of philosophy and sound physiology, so does the inspection of diseased and cachectic subjects powerfully assist philosophical pathology.[85]

Then, as now, physiology and pathology are separated in the medical curriculum. It was logical of Harvey to consider physiology first:

The physiological consideration . . . is to be first undertaken by medical men; since that which is in conformity with nature is right, and serves as a rule both to itself and to that which is amiss; by the light it sheds, too, aberrations and affections against nature are defined; pathology then stands out more clearly; and from pathology the use and art of healing, as well as occasions for the discovery of many new remedies, are perceived.[86]

Sound knowledge of pathology, he thought, was an essential foundation for the art of healing, and postmortem examinations revealed an extraordinary idea:

Nor could anyone really imagine how extensively internal organs are altered in diseases, especially chronic diseases, and what monstrosities among internal parts these diseases engender. So that I venture to say that the examination of a single body of one who has died of tabes or some other disease of long standing, or poisonous nature, is of more service to medicine than the dissection of the bodies of ten men who have been hanged.[87]

All physicians take for granted now that internal organs are altered in disease. Pathologists of today would still like to send this message to their colleagues: autopsies do add new information to medical science. All the technological wonders of modern diagnostic medicine have limitations on their sensitivity, specificity, precision, and predictive value. Looking at, and studying the tissues of, particular patients with known diseases continues to add to our understanding of these diseases and their treatments. These studies allow an objective look at the extent and nature of disease, the effects of treatment, and the possible basis for complications of the disease or its treatment. As more and more proposed, reference, or definitive molecular based methods arise (eg, DNA probes and monoclonal antibodies), it is important to test them in general application and at the same time, where possible, look at the internal structures of the cells of the various organs to see if new disease patterns can be discovered. Just as Harvey advocated looking into the body to observe organs altered in disease, medical scientists today are looking into the cells and subcellular molecular structures of cells to observe even more fundamental aspects of disease.

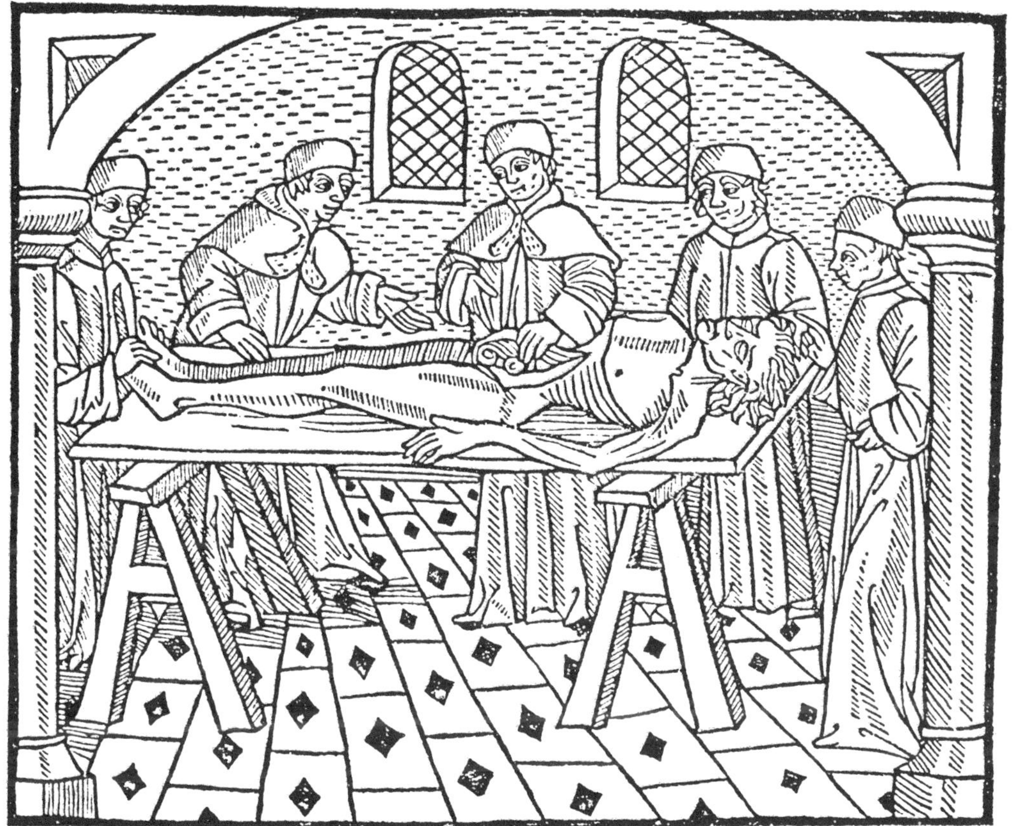

Through dissection, internal effects of disease are revealed.

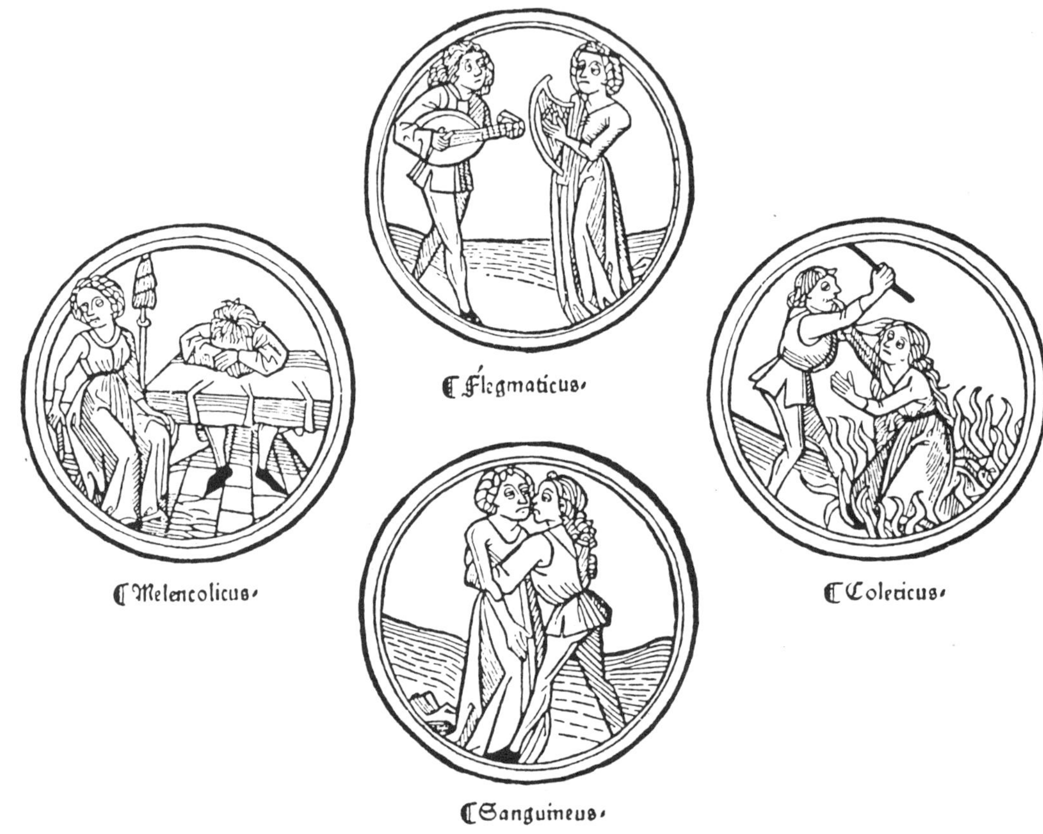

Flegmaticus.
Melencolicus.
Coleticus.
Sanguineus.

THE CATEGORIES OF DISEASE

13. Plato: Pain and Pleasure, Corruption and Inflammation

istorical philosophers tell us that Plato recounts observations, then questions if there is concurrence with the reigning philosophical constructs before espousing an opinion. Here follow some examples with medical relevance.

Plato tells us that disease and trauma lead to pain, but death itself may be painful or even pleasant:

> That which takes place according to nature is pleasant, but that which is contrary to nature is painful. And thus death, if caused by disease or produced by wounds, is painful and violent; but that sort of death which comes with old age and fulfils the debt of nature is the easiest of deaths, and is accompanied with pleasure rather than with pain.[88]

One wonders if the pneumonia we speak of as the old man's friend might not be fulfilling one of nature's debts.

Gangrene and tissue necrosis are not newly described processes:

> The oldest part of the flesh which is corrupted, being hard to decompose, from long burning grows black, and from being everywhere corroded becomes bitter, and is injurious to every part of the body which is still uncorrupted. Sometimes, when the bitter element is refined away, the black part assumes an acidity which takes the place of bitterness; at other times the bitterness being tinged with blood has a redder color; and this, when mixed with black, takes the hue of grass; and again, an auburn colour mingles with the bitter

matter when new flesh is decomposed by the fire which surrounds the internal flame—to all which symptoms some physician perhaps, or rather some philosopher, who had the power of seeing in many dissimilar things one nature deserving of a name, has assigned the common name of bile.[89]

Could the biochemical engines that produce adenosine triphosphate (ATP) be our modern equivalent of the "internal flame?"

Bodily excretions not cleared or stress induced by starvation or fluid deprivation could have dire consequences:

Decomposition of tender flesh when intermingled with air is termed by us white phlegm. And the whey or sediment of newly formed phlegm is sweat and tears, and includes the various daily discharges by which the body is purified. Now all these become causes of disease when the blood is not replenished in a natural manner by food and drink but gains bulk from opposite sources in violation of the laws of nature.[90]

Internal abnormalities rather than external or environmental effects could also in Plato's era, it was thought, lead to disease:

There is [another] . . . class of diseases which may be conceived of as arising in three ways; for they are produced sometimes by wind and sometimes by phlegm and sometimes by bile. When the lung . . . is obstructed by rheums . . . then the parts which are unrefreshed by air corrode . . . [or] in other parts excess of air forcing its way through the veins distorts them . . . and the body is enclosed in the midst of it . . . . Thus numberless painful diseases are produced, accompanied by copious sweats . . . . The greatest pain is felt when the wind gets about the sinews and the veins of the shoulders, and swells them up. . . . These disorders are called tetanus and opisthotonus by reason of the tension which accompanies them.[91]

Today we do not think of air as circulating in veins, but we do know that diaphoresis occurs in numerous conditions, infectious and otherwise.

Inflammatory processes can affect any and all portions of the body. Plato seems to have concentrated on the fever that is present in such cases and to have attributed it to bilious excess:

Inflammations of the body come from burnings and inflamings, and all of them originate in bile. When bile finds a means of discharge, it boils up and sends forth all sorts of tumours; but when imprisoned within, it generates many inflammatory diseases, above all when mingled with pure blood. . . . If it [bile] have power enough to maintain its supremacy, it penetrates the marrow and burns up what may be termed the cables of the soul, and sets her free; but when there is not so much of it, and the body, though wasted, still holds out, the bile is itself mastered, and is either utterly banished, or is thrust through the veins into the lower or upper belly, and is driven out of the body like an exile from a state in which there has been a civil war whence arise diarrhoeas and dysenteries, and all such disorders.[92]

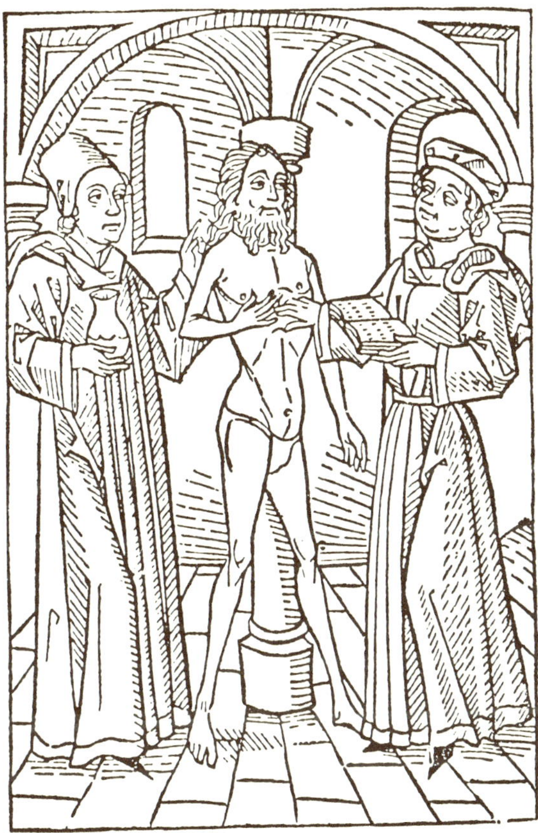

The physician observes, examines, and looks to his books for concurrence.

♦ 57 ♦

Centuries later, Rudolph Virchow posited a
"civil war" between cellular elements of the body
as one way of conceiving of disease processes. We
to this day talk about autoimmune disorders—for
example, systemic lupus erythematosus—as examples of self-destruction of the organism by ab-
normal immunocytes whose cells or products
attack the affected patient's own tissues.

14. Hippocrates: Seasons, Winds, and Skull Fractures

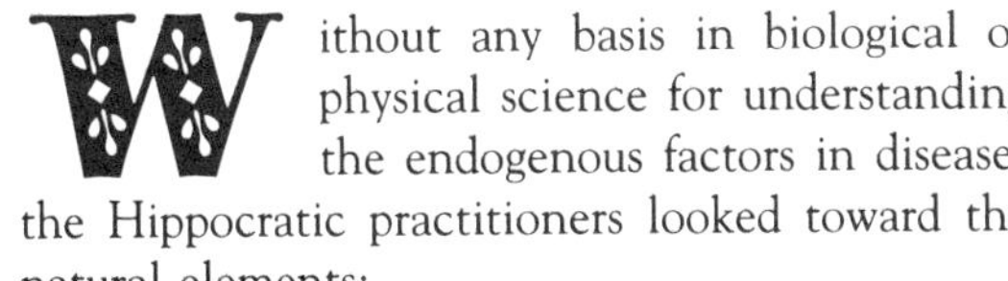

ithout any basis in biological or physical science for understanding the endogenous factors in disease, the Hippocratic practitioners looked toward the natural elements:

[In] a city that is exposed to hot winds . . . but which is sheltered from the north winds . . . the heads of the inhabitants are of a humid and pituitous constitution, and their bellies subject to frequent disorders, owing to the phlegm running down from the head; the forms of their bodies, for the most part, are rather flabby. . . . The following diseases are peculiar to the district: in the first place, the women are sickly and subject to excessive menstruation; then many are unfruitful from disease, and not from nature, and they have frequent miscarriages; infants are subject to attacks of convulsions and asthma, which they consider to be connected with infancy, and hold to be a sacred disease (epilepsy). The men are subject to attacks of dysentery, diarrhea, hepialus, chronic fevers in winter, of epinyctis, frequently, and of hemorrhoids about the anus. . . . If any epidemic disease connected with the change of seasons prevail, they are also liable to it.[93]

Not only the nature of the disease but the severity of the affliction would vary by site:

[In] cities that are exposed to winds between the summer and the winter risings of the sun . . . the persons of the inhabitants are, for the most part, well colored and blooming, unless some disease counteract. . . . Diseases are few in number, and of a feeble kind, and bear a resemblance to the diseases which prevail in regions exposed to hot winds. The women there are very prolific, and have easy deliveries.[94]

But such cities as lie to the west, and which are sheltered from winds blowing from the east, and which the hot winds and the cold winds of the north scarcely touch, must necessarily be in a very unhealthy situation: in the first place the waters are not clear, the cause of which is because the mist prevails commonly in the morning, and it is mixed up with the water and destroys its clearness. . . . The inhabitants . . . are pale and enfeebled.[95]

The malevolvent nature of unclear (contaminated) water is a recurrent theme:

Water contributes much towards health. . . . Waters then as are marshy, stagnant, and belong to lakes . . . are unwholesome and form bile. . . . They are most apt to engender phlegm, and bring on hoarseness; those who drink them have large and obstructed spleens, their bellies are hard, emaciated and hot; and their shoulders, collar-bones, and faces are emaciated; for their flesh is melted down and taken up by the spleen, and hence they are slender; such persons then are voracious and thirsty; their bellies are very dry both above and below, so that they require the strongest medicines. . . . They are very subject to dropsies of a most fatal character; and in summer dysenteries, diarrheas, and protracted quartan fevers frequently seize them. . . . In winter younger persons are liable to pneumonia and maniacal affections; and older persons to ardent fevers, from hardness of the belly. Women are subject to oedema and lecophlegmasiae; when pregnant they have difficult deliveries; their infants are large and swelled, and then during nursing they become wasted and sickly, and the lochial discharge after parturition does not proceed properly with the women. The children are particularly subject to hernia, and adults to varices and ulcers on their legs.[96]

Except for epidemics, a few acute diseases were taught to be the most common causes of death:

> Acute diseases are those which the ancients named pleurisy, pneumonia, phrenitis, lethargy, causus, and the other diseases allied to these, including the continual fevers. For, unless when some general form of pestilential disease is epidemic, and diseases are sporadic and (not) of a similar character, there are more deaths from these diseases than from all the others taken together.[97]

We still advise students of medicine to be meticulous in history taking, to pay attention to detail:

> With regard to diseases, the circumstances from which we form a judgment of them are—by attending to the general nature of all, and the peculiar nature of each individual; to the disease, the patient, and the applications; to the person who applies them, as that makes a difference for better or for worse; to the whole constitution of the season, and particularly to the state of the heavens and the nature of each country; to the patient's habits, regimen, and pursuits; to his conversation, manners, taciturnity, thoughts, sleep, or absence of sleep, and sometimes his dreams, what and when they occur; to his picking and scratching; to his tears; to the alvine discharges, urine, sputa, and vomitings; and to the changes of diseases from the one into the other; to the sweat, coldness, rigor, cough, sneezing, hiccup, respiration, eructation, flatulence, whether passed silently or with a noise; to hemorrhages and hemorrhoids; from these, and their consequences, we must form our judgment. Fevers are the continual, some of which hold during the day and have a remission at night, and others hold during the night and have a remission during the day; semi-tertians, tertians, quartans, quintans, septans, nonans. The most acute, strongest, most dangerous, and fatal diseases occur in the continual fever. The least dangerous of all, and the mildest and most protracted, is the quartan.[98]

Nowadays, we look for an underlying cause of fever. The ancients only had the patient and the fever; so great care was given to characterizing the fever and distinguishing among patients based on the many variations in this sign:

The nocturnal fever is not very fatal, but protracted; the diurnal is still more protracted, and in some cases passes into phthisis. . . .[99]

There are peculiar modes, and constitutions, and paroxysms, in every one of these fevers; for example, the continual, in some cases at the very commencement, grows, as it were, and attains its full strength, and rises to its most dangerous pitch, but is diminished about and at the crisis; in others it begins gentle and suppressed, but gains ground and is exacerbated every day, and bursts forth with all its heat about and at the crisis; while in others, again, it commences mildly, increases, and is exacerbated until it reaches its acme, and then remits until at and about the crisis. These varieties occur in every fever, and in every disease.

From these observations one must regulate the regimen accordingly.[100]

For the peripatetic physician, the Hippocratic school offers some good advice:

Whoever wishes to investigate medicine properly should proceed thus: in the first place to consider the seasons of the year, and what effects each of them produces, for they are not all alike, but differ much from themselves in regard to their changes. . . . Then the winds . . . the qualities of the waters . . . the situation of the city. . . . For if one knows all these things well, or at least the greater part of them, he cannot miss knowing, when he comes into a strange city, either the diseases peculiar to the place, or the particular nature of common diseases.[101]

In *Injuries of the Head,* there is an uncannily perceptive description of the various types of head trauma.

1. When a wounded bone breaks, in the bone comprehending the fissure, contusion necessarily takes place where the bone is broken. . . .

2. . . . A bone may be contused, and yet remain in its natural condition without any fracture in it. . . .

3. . . . The bone being fractured is sometimes depressed inwards from its natural level along with the fractures, otherwise there would be no depression, for the depressed portion being fractured and broken off, is pushed inwards, while the rest of the bone remains in its natural position; and in this manner a fracture is combined with the depression.

4. When a hedra, or dint of a weapon, takes place in a bone, there may be a fracture combined with it; and provided there be a fracture, contusion must necessarily be joined, to a greater or less extent, in the seat of the dint and fracture, and in the bone which comprehends them.

5. A bone may be injured in a different part of the head from that on which the person has received the wound. . . . For this misfortune, when it occurs, there is no remedy; for when this mischief takes place, there is no means of ascertaining by any examination whether or not it has occurred, or on what part of the head.[102]

The accuracy of some of these guidelines most likely flows from their observational base; that is, these guidelines derive from the collected experiences of practitioners in particular patients in similar circumstances. Detailed observations were doubtlessly made and recorded on seriously injured patients who may have received a great deal of attention. In contrast to more general speculation about the possible effects of seasons or temperature on the occurrence of disease in a population, in these five rules specific, definite correlations between the nature of the wound, the way of wounding, and the disrupted anatomical structures are recorded.

Conflicting approaches to the management of trauma are not new:

The greater part of physicians treat fractures, both with and without an external wound, during the first days, by means of unwashed wool, and there does not appear to be anything improper in this. . . . [One of the] most important principles of medicine: . . . at no time is it so little proper to disturb all kinds of wounds as on the third and fourth day; and all sort of probing should be avoided on these days in whatever other injuries are attended with irritation. For, generally, the third and fourth day, in most cases of wounds, are those which give rise to exacerbations, whether the tendency be to inflammation, to a foul condition of the sore, or to fevers.[103]

Some of the ancient observations on bones and joints represent a basic common-sense approach:

In a word, luxations and subluxations take place in different degrees, being sometimes greater and sometimes less; and those cases in which the bone has slipped or been displaced to a much greater extent, are in general more difficult to rectify than otherwise; and if not reduced, such cases have greater and more striking impairment and lesion of the bones, fleshy parts, and attitudes; but when the bone has slipped, or been displaced to a less extent it is easier to reduce such cases than the other; and if the attempts at reduction have failed, or have been neglected, the impairment in such cases is less, and proves less injurious than in the cases just mentioned.[104]

Anatomy, then as now, was the foundation of good surgery:

The heads of the femur and humerus are very similar to one another as to their dislocations. For the heads of the bones are rounded and smooth, and the sockets which receive the heads are also circular, and adapted to the heads.[105]

Orthopedics, the surgical specialty originally devoted to the restoration of function by straightening the arms and legs of children, goes back many centuries, as evidenced by this ancient advice on treating clubfoot:

Most cases of congenital club foot are remediable, unless the declination be very great, or when the affection occurs at an advanced period of youth. The best plan, then, is to treat such cases at as early a

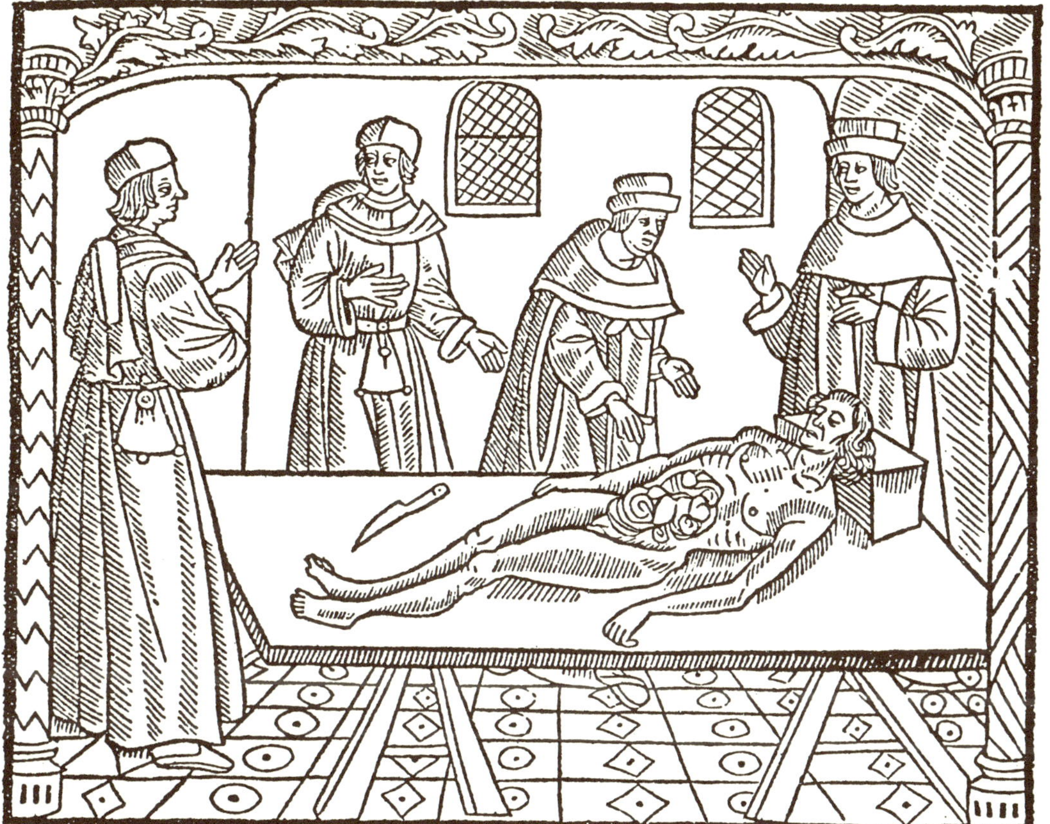

Ancient observations are
the bases of many regimens
of modern medicine.

period as possible, before the deficiency of the bones of the foot is very great, and before there is any great wasting of the flesh of the leg.[106]

The Hippocratic aphorisms contain many interesting and still pertinent observations. Much of their thrust is toward the environment and effects of the elements on human health:

5. South winds induce dullness of hearing, dimness of visions, heaviness of the head, torpor, and languor; when these prevail, such symptoms occur in diseases. But if the north wind prevail, coughs, affections of the throat, hardness of the bowels, dysuria attended with rigors, and pains of the sides and breast occur. When this wind prevails, all such symptoms may be expected in diseases.[107]

As nature slows down for winter, those in decline may be more at risk:

9. In autumn, diseases are most acute, and most mortal, on the whole. The spring is most healthy, and least mortal.[108]

The following statements may have related to insect-borne disease, especially the fevers:

15. Of the constitutions of the year, the dry, upon the whole, are more healthy than the rainy, and attended with less mortality.

16. The diseases which occur most frequently in rainy seasons are protracted fevers, fluxes of the bowels, mortifications, epilepsies, apoplexies, and quinsies; and in dry consumptive diseases, ophthalmies, arthritic diseases, stranguries, and dysenteries.[109]

Seasons of the year are not so pervasively important in modern patient data bases as they were in the Hippocratic era, but the admonitions and descriptions are interesting to review. In allergic disorders and some infectious diseases, seasonality is quite real, definite, and reproducible.

19. All diseases occur at all seasons of the year, but certain of them are more apt to occur and be exacerbated at certain seasons.

20. The diseases of spring are maniacal,
melancholic, and epileptic disorders,
bloody flux, quinsy, coryza, hoarseness,
cough, leprosy, lichen alphos,
exanthemata mostly ending in ulcerations,
tubercles, and arthritic diseases.

The coryza and cough could well have related to molds and pollens in the air causing allergic reactions such as hay fever.

21. Of autumn, most of the summer,
quartan, and irregular fevers, enlarged
spleen, dropsy, phthisis, strangury,
lientery, dysentery, sciatica, quinsy,
asthma, ileus, epilepsy, maniacal and
melancholic disorders.

23. Of winter, pleurisy, pneumonia,
coryza, pains, hoarseness, cough of the
chest, pains of the ribs and loins,
headache, vertigo, and apoplexy.[110]

Some of these winter diseases with cold and chest symptoms and aches and pains likely did represent seasonal afflictions from viral infections that we still observe in influenza, for example.

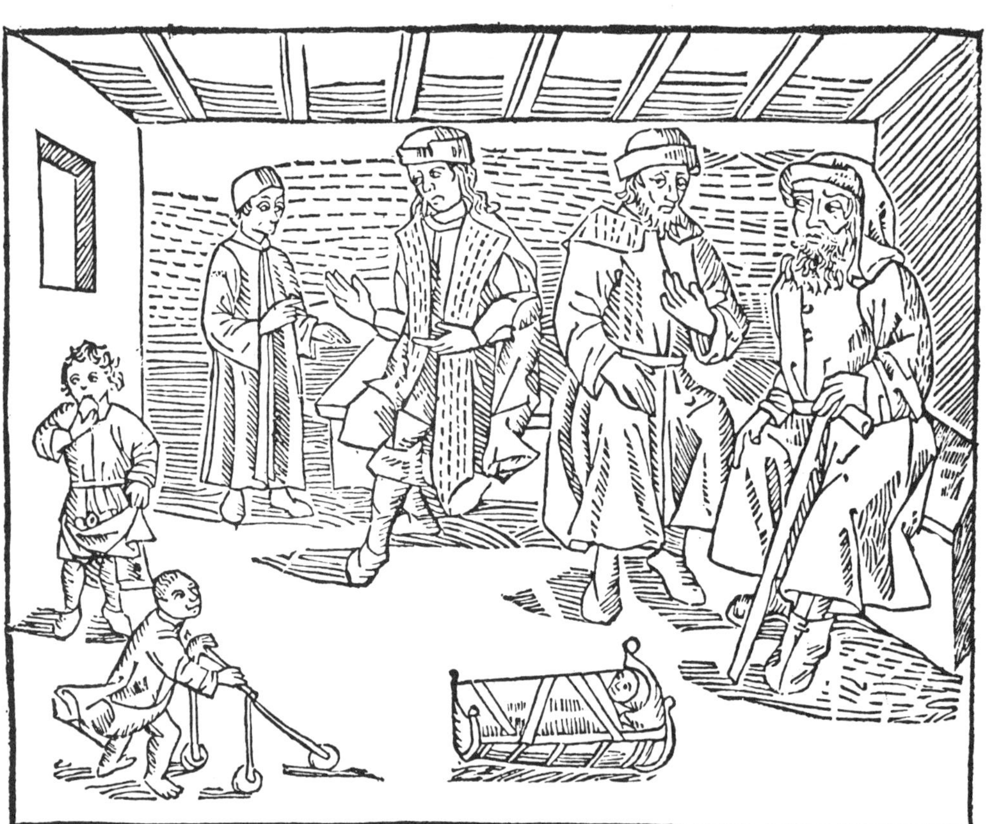

THE NATURAL HISTORY
OF DISEASE

15. Old Testament: The Dreaded Skin Disease

The Old Testament, in Leviticus 13:15, gives a quite ancient perspective on dermatology. Some lesions could become severe, others not. The patient had to submit to a ritual examination to determine the proper course of action under laws concerning skin diseases and unclean bodily discharges.

If anyone has a sore on his skin or a boil or an inflammation which could develop into a dreaded skin disease, he shall be brought to the Aaronite priest. The priest shall examine the sore, and if the hairs in it have turned white and the sore appears to be deeper than the surrounding skin, it is a dreaded skin disease, and the priest shall pronounce the person unclean. But if the sore is white and does not appear to be deeper than the skin around it and the hairs have not turned white, the priest shall isolate the person for seven days.[111]

The color of the hair, perhaps signifying necrosis or death of the hair bulbs, is important in skin lesions.

If anyone has a dreaded skin disease, he shall be brought to the priest who will examine him. If there is a white sore on his skin which turns the hairs white and is full of pus, it is a chronic skin disease. . . . If the skin disease spreads and covers the person from head to foot . . . [and] if his whole skin has turned white, he is ritually clean. But from the moment an open sore appears, he is unclean.[112]

Aristotle comments on only a few particular signs associated with particular diseases. Like the Old Testament, *On the Generation of Animals* gives a specific detail helpful in diagnosis of a dreaded ancient skin disease.

In what is called leprosy the hairs become white.[113]

We now know that this sign is not diagnostic of *Mycobacterium leprae* infection; but then many chronic inflammatory dermatoses and other lesions were traditionally lumped together as leprosy when, in fact, probably only a modest fraction were the actual disease caused by Hansen's bacillus (*M. leprae*).

Gonorrhea is also an age-old disease.

When any man has a discharge from his penis, the discharge is unclean, whether the penis runs with it or is stopped up by it. Any bed upon which he sits or lies is unclean . . . anyone who touches his bed . . . must wash his clothes and take a bath.[114]

In those days the rules were stricter; the breaking of a quarantine could have fatal consequences:

The Lord told Moses to warn the people of Israel about their uncleanness, so that they would not defile the Tent of his presence. . . . If they did they would be killed.[115]

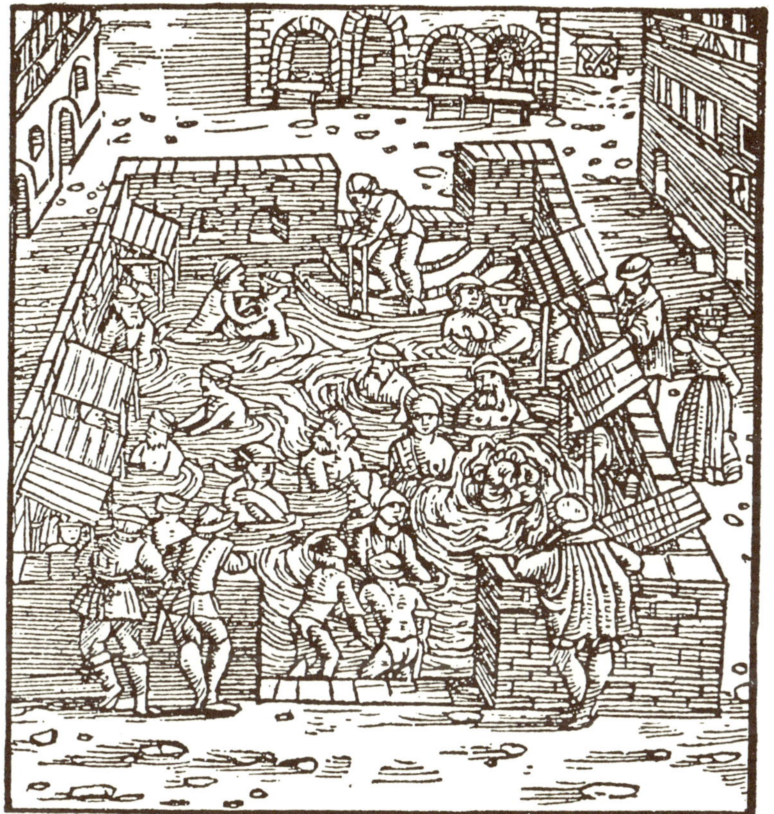

Bathing has always been a healthful (and sometimes sanitary) practice.

16. Thucydides: The Peloponnesian War and the Plague of Athens

Thucydides' description of the devastating plague of Athens, which affected the outcome of the Peloponnesian War, is just now being understood. A recent article by twentieth-century infectious disease specialists argues that this epidemic was influenza followed by bacterial infection (probably staphylococcal) similar to toxic shock syndrome.[116]

Read this masterful description of what happened to the doctors and patients.

Neither were the physicians at first of any service, ignorant as they were of the proper way to treat it, but they died themselves the most thickly, as they visited the sick most often. . . .

As a rule there was . . . no ostensible cause; but people in good health were all of a sudden attacked by violent heats in the head, and redness and inflammation in the eyes, the inward parts, such as the throat or tongue, becoming bloody and emitting an unnatural and fetid breath . . . followed by sneezing and hoarseness, after which pain soon reached the chest, and produced a hard cough. . . . When it fixed in the stomach it upset it; and discharges of bile of every kind named by physicians ensued, accompanied by great distress. . . . The disease descended further into the bowels, inducing a violent ulceration accompanied by severe diarrhea, this brought on a weakness which was generally fatal. . . . Others again were

seized with an entire loss of memory on
their first recovery, and did not know
either themselves or their friends. Strong
and weak constitutions proved equally
incapable of resistance. . . . By far the
most terrible feature in the malady was the
dejection which ensued when any one felt
himself sickening, for the despair into
which they instantly fell took away their
power of resistance, and left them a much
easier prey to the disorder. . . .

[T]here was the awful spectacle of men
dying like sheep, through having caught
the infection in nursing each other. . . .
Honour made them unsparing of
themselves in their attendance in their
friends' houses. . . . Yet it was with those
who had recovered from the disease that
the sick and dying found most compassion.
These knew what it was from experience,
and had now no fear for themselves; for
the same man was never attacked twice—
never at least fatally. And such persons
. . . half entertained the vain hope that
they were for the future safe from any
disease whatsoever.[117]

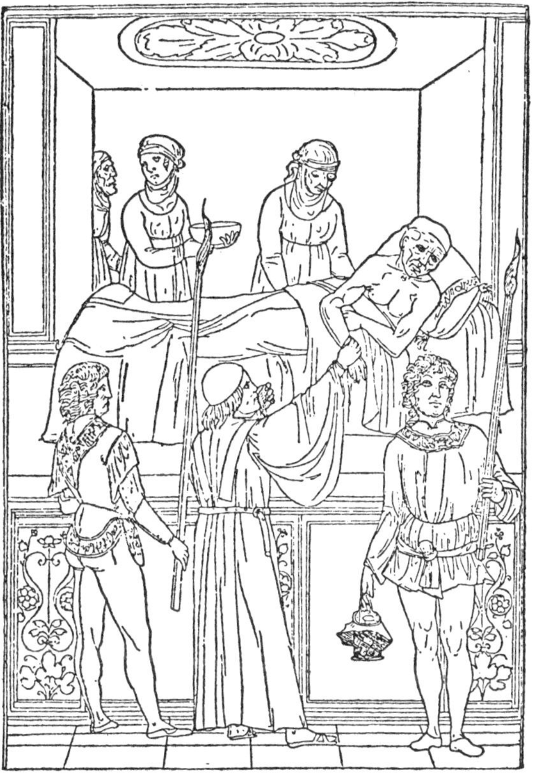

This observation on protection from a second attack raises the question of how well or widely the principle of immunity might have been understood at that time. It was not until many centuries later that Edward Jenner demonstrated the technique of artificial immunization by vaccine. Here the protection was from the natural disease and certainly was understood and believed in well enough to allow survivors to be the ones who preferentially provided care for subsequent victims. Perhaps the hope that prior affliction and survival of this plague protected against any disease resembles the associative thought process in persons today who demand penicillin for a viral infection. If it's good for streptococcal sore throat, it must be good for all sore throats!

17. Hippocrates: Prognosis

In *The Book of Prognostics* we read some very sage advice: It is impossible to make all the sick well.[118] In this day of lawsuits, defensive practice, and emerging distrust between doctors and patients, it would be well for doctors, patients, and attorneys to recall this bit of wisdom.

Doctors are well advised to know their patients, inside and out, for medical and practical reasons relating to risk management.

> It therefore becomes necessary to know the
> nature of such affections, how far they are
> above the powers of the constitution. . . .
> Thus a man will be the more esteemed to
> be a good physician, for he will be the
> better able to treat those aright who can
> be saved, from having long anticipated
> everything; and by seeing and announcing
> beforehand those who will live and those
> who will die, he will thus escape
> censure.[119]

Unlikely it is that all physicians will escape censure. Yet thoroughness is certainly a desirable trait in the medical doctor.

Some of the signs important to the Hippocratic physicians are still quite significant and heeded to this day:

> The worst [prognosis is indicated by] . . .
> a sharp nose, hollow eyes, collapsed
> temples; the ears cold, contracted, and
> their lobes turned out; the skin about the
> forehead being rough, distended, and
> parched; the color of the whole face being
> green, black, livid, or lead-colored.[120]

Others do not seem so valid:

It is well when the patient is found by his physician reclining upon either his right or his left side. . . . But to lie upon one's back, with the hands, neck, and the legs extended, is far less favorable.[121]

Those dealing with neurologically impaired patients would be likely interested in this ancient observation:

When in acute fevers . . . the hands are waved before the face, hunting through empty space, as if gathering bits of straw, picking the nap from the coverlet, or tearing chaff from the wall—all such symptoms are bad and deadly.[122]

Tachypnea was appreciated as serious:

Respiration, when frequent, indicates pain or inflammation in the parts above the diaphragm.[123]

So was acute peripheral edema:

All dropsies arising from acute diseases are bad.[124]

Some of the current teaching about shock—hypovolemic and septic—had forerunners in ancient times.

It is a bad symptom when the head, hands, and feet are cold, while the belly and sides are hot; but it is a very good symptom when the whole body is equally hot.[125]

Modern laboratory medicine can generate many analyses on the various body specimens; sometimes we are tempted to lose sight of the significant observations the physician can make at the bedside.

The excrement is best which is soft and consistent, is passed at the hour which was customary to the patient when in health. . . but excrements that are very watery, or white, or green, or very red, or frothy, are all bad. It is also bad when the discharge is small and viscid, and white, and greenish, and smooth; but still more deadly appearances are the black, or fatty, or livid, or verdigris-green, or fetid.[126]

Macroscopic urinalysis has been superseded by

microscopic and biochemical studies; but how many physicians of today actually take a look at fluid specimens themselves? If they did, the following might be confirmed as accurate:

> The urine is best when the sediment is white, smooth, and consistent during the whole time.[127]

Hematemesis is a serious sign now as then:

> But if that which is vomited be of the color of leeks or livid, or black, whatever of these colors it be, it is to be reckoned bad.[128]

Some old observations about the color of sputum and about breath sounds in what we now call pneumonia still have validity.

> Expectoration . . . should be quickly and easily brought up, and a certain degree of yellowness should appear . . . but ruddy color is worse; . . . that which is intensely yellow is dangerous, . . . that which is very green and frothy is bad; but if so intense as to appear black, it is still more dangerous . . .; it is bad if nothing is expectorated, and the lungs discharge nothing, but are gorged with matters which boil (as it were) in the air passages.[129]

Parts of this description of empyema (acute inflammation of the space surrounding the lung, usually infectious) are still valid:

> Empyema may be recognized in all cases by the following symptoms: In the first place, the fever does not go off, but is slight during the day, and increases at night, and copious sweats supervene, there is a desire to cough, and the patients expectorate nothing worth mentioning, the eyes become hollow, the cheeks have red spots on them, the nails of the hands are bent, the fingers are hot—especially their extremities, there are swellings in the feet, they have no desire of food, and small blisters (phlyctaenae) occur over the body.[130]

Acute urinary retention is still an emergency:

> When the bladder is hard and painful, it is an extremely bad and mortal

symptom. . . . Urine of a purulent character relieves the patient. . . . This form attacks children more especially, from their seventh to their fifteenth year.[131]

This description of headache and fever is quite general but likely did predict the outcome of some cases of bacterial meningitis:

> Strong and continued headaches with fever, if any of the deadly symptoms be joined to them, are very fatal.[132]

Particularly deadly symptoms included acute urinary obstruction and difficult respiration. A similar outcome also followed upon some cases of acute otitis media in which meningitis probably developed.

> Acute pain of the ear, with continual and strong fever, is to be dreaded; for there is danger that the man may become delirious and die.[133]

Maintaining an airway is critical in conditions that compromise the flow of air into the trachea. In an earlier era, a now readily treated infection could well lead to serious consequences for the patient:

Ulceration of the throat with fever is a serious affection. . . . Those quinsies are most dangerous, and most quickly prove fatal, which make no appearance in the fauces, nor in the neck, but occasion very great pain and difficulty of breathing; these induce suffocation on the first day, or on the second, the third, or the fourth.[134]

Wise would be the physician who could always accurately predict disease outcome; but with a good history, physical examination, laboratory studies, and epidemiological considerations a doctor at least has a reasonable chance:

> He who would know correctly beforehand those that will recover, and those that will die, and in what cases the disease will be protracted for many days, and in what cases for a shorter time, must be able to form a judgment from having made himself acquainted with all the symptoms, and estimating their powers in comparison with one another, as has been described, with regard to the others, and the urine and sputa, as when the patient coughs up pus and bile together. One ought to consider

promptly the influx of epidemical
diseases. . . . One should . . . be well
acquainted with the particular signs and
the other symptoms, and not be ignorant
how that, in every year, and at every
season, bad symptoms prognosticate ill,
and favorable symptoms good. [135]

In *On Regimen in Acute Diseases*, we learn
about the importance of historical details.

[The physician should] mark, particularly,
the first day on which the patient became
ill, considering when and whence the
disease commenced. [136]

A *comprehensive* medical history is essential to
each patient's evaluation:

When you examine the patient, inquire
into all particulars. [137]

This observation is too inclusive; nonetheless,
there is some accuracy to it regarding infectious
diseases:

All diseases are resolved either by the
mouth, the bowels, the bladder, or some
other such organ. Sweat is a common form
of resolution. [138]

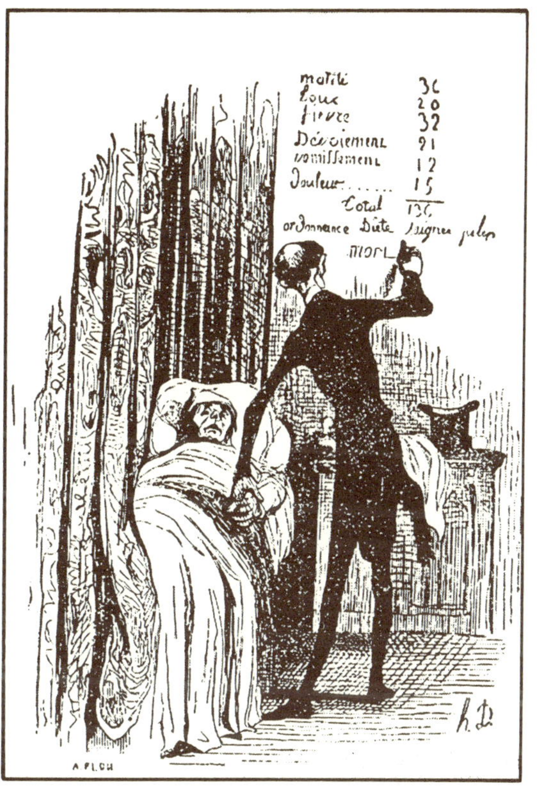

Sometimes Fate tallies the best prognosis.

Infectious diseases were the most prevalent form of serious acute illness:

> The most important point of regimen to observe, and be guarded about in protracted diseases, is to pay attention to the exacerbations and remissions of fevers.[139]

In *On Injuries of the Head*, we get a clinical picture of the serious consequences of an open head wound in the pre-antibiotic era.

> When a person has sustained a mortal wound on the head, which cannot be cured, nor his life preserved, you may form an opinion of his approaching dissolution, and foretell what is to happen from the following symptoms which such a person experiences. When a bone is broken, or cleft, or contused, or otherwise injured, and when by mistake it has not been discovered, and neither the raspatory nor trepan has been applied as required, but the case has been neglected as if the bone were sound, fever will generally come on before the fourteenth day if in winter, and in summer the fever usually seizes after seven days. And when this happens, the wound loses its color, and the inflammation dies in it; and it becomes glutinous, and appears like a pickle, being of a tawny and somewhat livid color; and the bone then begins to sphacelate, and it turns black where it was white before, and at last becomes pale and blanched. But when suppuration is fairly established in it, small blisters form on the tongue and he dies delirious.[140]

In serious intracranial lesions we now know the anatomical basis for these ancient observations:

> And, for the most part, convulsions seize the other side of the body; for, if the wound be situated on the left side, the convulsions will seize the right side of the body; or if the wound be situated on the left side, the convulsions will seize the right side of the body. . . . And some become apoplectic. And thus they die before the end of seven days, if in summer; and before fourteen if in winter.[141]

18. Lucretius: Mind, Body, and Miasm

In *On the Nature of Things*, we learn about some postulated interactions between mind and body in cases of severe illness that remind us of some of the writings of Plato.

Even as the body is liable to violent diseases and severe pain, so is the mind to sharp cares and grief and fear; it naturally follows therefore that it is its partner in death as well . . . . In diseases of the body the mind often wanders and goes astray; for it loses its reason, drivels in its speech, and often in a profound lethargy is carried into deep and never-ending sleep.[142]

Epilepsy is a frequent subject for ancient philosphical-medical discourse. The abrupt onset of a seizure with loss of function was, and still is, a frightening event, especially for those who do not understand the disease.

It often happens that some one constrained by the violence of disease suddenly drops down before our eyes, as by a stroke of lightning, and foams at the mouth, moans and shivers through his frame, loses his reason, stiffens his muscles, is racked, gasps for breath fitfully. . . . Then after the cause of the disease has bent its course back and the acrid humours of the distempered body return to their hiding places, then he first gets up like one reeling, and by little and little comes back into full possession of his senses and regains his soul.[143]

Bad air, as in malaria, was often considered

the cause of what are now known to be parasitic diseases:

> There is the elephant disease which is generated beside the streams of the Nile in the midst of Egypt and nowhere else. In Attica the feet are attacked and the eyes in Achaean lands. And so different places are hurtful to different parts and members: the variations of air occasion that . . . this . . . destroying power and pestilence therefore all at once either fall upon the waters or else sink deep into the corn-crops or other food of man . . . or else their force remains suspended within the atmosphere, and when we inhale from it mixed airs, we must absorb at the same time into our body those things as well.[144]

The danger of bad air as described here reminds us of the importance placed upon winds, seasons, and climates by Hippocrates. Many persons to this day still emphasize the importance of fresh air, especially while sleeping, to good health. The philosopher gives us another example of a severe disease related to noxious, in this case, foreign, atmosphere:

> A form of disease and a death-fraught miasm . . . rising first from Egypt . . . after traversing much air . . . brooded over the whole people [who] first of all . . . would have the head seized with burning heat and both eyes blood-shot with a glare diffused over. . . . The livid throat within would exude blood and the passage of the voice be clogged and choked with ulcers . . . when the force of disease passing down the throat had filled the breast and had streamed together even into the sad heart of the sufferers, then would all the barriers of life give way.[145]

In the last two instances, bad air is given as the cause of fatal disease. We now know that elephantiasis is related to parasites living in bad water, not to inhalation of bad air. Perhaps these waters are the unclear ones pronounced dangerous by Hippocrates. The febrile illness could have been diphtheria or another infectious disease—in any event, not one caused by bad air. It is striking, in light of what we now know about the cardiac damaging effects of toxins from some strains of diphtheria, that Lucretius pointed out the special effects of this particular overwhelming disease upon the heart of the sufferer.

We now know and better understand how severe pain and diseases of the brain and heart can cause pathophysiological dysfunctions. We know they can be disspiriting or disheartening as, in the latter two cases, they lead to seizures or cardiac failure. Lucretius tells us that there are definite interactions between mind and body, between emotional status and disease state. We still face this reality every day in twentieth-century medicine.

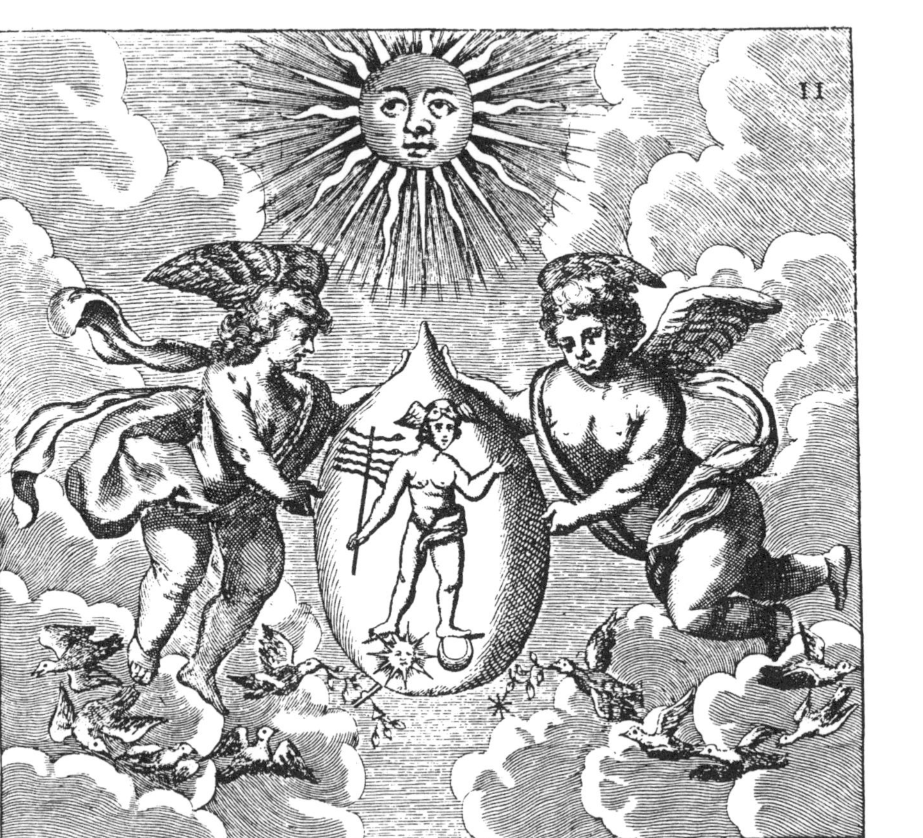

THE CAUSES OF DISEASE 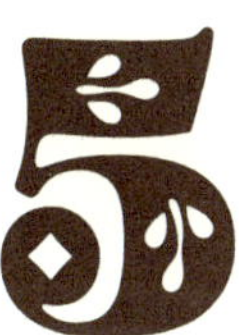

PART 5

19. Old Testament, Apocrypha, and New Testament: Punishment and Exorcism

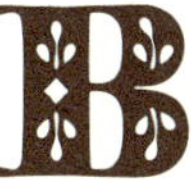efore medicine developed as a separate profession, as recorded in the Old Testament, the priests were responsible for most health issues and developed elaborate purification rituals to deal with diseases. Disease is presented with an emphasis on the personal, spiritual relationships between the afflicted and God. In these examples from the Pentateuch, God's punishment for willful disobedience is a leading cause of disease.

> I will punish you. I will bring disaster on you—incurable diseases and fevers that will make you blind and cause your life to waste away.[146]

> The Lord was angry with them; and so as he departed and the cloud left the tent, Miriam's skin was suddenly covered with a dreaded disease and turned as white as snow. When Aaron looked at her and saw that she was covered with the disease, he said to Moses, "Please, sir, do not make us suffer this punishment for our foolish sin. Don't let her become like something born dead with half its flesh eaten away."[147]

This interpretation applied to epidemics as well as isolated cases:

> Moses said to Aaron, "Take your fire pan, put live coals from the altar in it, and put some incense on the coals. Then hurry with it to the people and perform the ritual of purification for them. Hurry! The Lord's anger has already broken out and an epidemic has already begun." Aaron obeyed, took his fire pan and ran into the

middle of the assembled people. When he
saw that the plague had already begun, he
put the incense on the coals and performed
the ritual of purification for the people.
This stopped the plague, and he was left
standing between the living and the dead.
The number of people who died was
14,700, not counting those who died in
Korah's rebellion.[148]

Infections were a common form of disease attributed to divine retribution in the Bible.

> If you do evil and reject the Lord . . . He
> will send disease after disease on you until
> there is not one of you left in the land
> that you are about to occupy. The Lord
> will strike you with infectious diseases,
> with swelling and fever.[149]

Besides the lesion, a large element of suffering was also attributed to the punishment. The retribution was so strong and pervasive in some instances that not only was there the affliction, even worse, there was no hope of cure.

> The Lord will send boils on you, as he did
> on the Egyptians. He will make your
> bodies break out with sores. You will be
> covered with scabs, and you will itch, but
> there will be no cure.[150]

Mental ills as well as physical came under the same rubric:

> The Lord will make you lose your mind;
> he will strike you with blindness and
> confusion.[151]

Not only were individuals to be afflicted; their heirs and descendants were not free from harm.

> The Lord will cover your legs with
> incurable, painful sores; boils will cover
> you from head to foot. . . . He will send
> on you and on your descendants incurable
> diseases and horrible epidemics that can
> never be stopped.[152]

One despised ruler was stricken with what seems to be a severe acute intestinal obstruction:

> The Lord struck [Antiochus] . . . down
> with an invisible but fatal blow. He was
> seized with sharp intestinal pains for which
> there was no relief—a fitting punishment
> for the man who had tortured others in so

many terrible ways. . . . He fell flat on
the ground.[153]

In this case, it also seems, the processes of postmortem decomposition and decay extended into
life. Wormy infestation of necrotic tissues by fly
larvae (myiasis) is one possibility. (Onchocer-
ciasis or eye worm parasite seems less likely in the
Levant than it would have been in Africa.) The
odor indicates that there was extensive tissue
damage with probable extensive bacterial over-
growth.

> Even the eyes of this godless man were
> crawling with worms and he lived in
> terrible pain and agony. The stink was so
> bad that his entire army was sickened.[154]

The New Testament concentrates more on examples of Jesus' healing of ill persons than on the
diseases themselves; but there are a few commentaries on the cause of disease, usually attributed
to possession by demons. In the gospel according
to Matthew, we hear about such a case.

> Some people brought to Jesus a man who
> could not talk because he had a demon.
> But as soon as the demon was driven out,

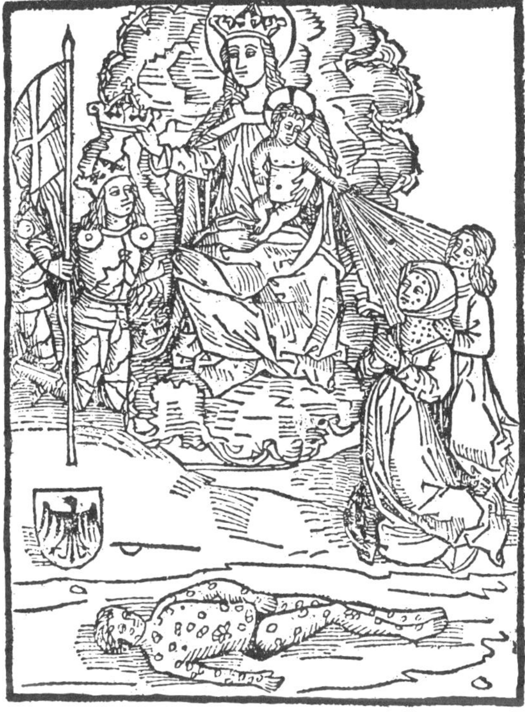

An allegory of epidemic
syphilis shows a holy hand
casting forth the scourge.

the man started talking and everyone was amazed.[155]

And another:

A man came to Jesus . . . and said, "Sir, have mercy on my son! He is an epileptic and has such terrible fits that he often falls into the fire or water. . . . Jesus gave a command to the demon, and it went out of the body, and at that very moment he was healed.[156]

Later in the New Testament, Paul attributes some of the afflictions of early Christians to their failure to understand the meaning of the spiritual aspect of eating and drinking in communion. Because of their profaning of a sacred moment, they come under God's judgment:

For if he does not recognize the meaning of the Lord's body when he eats the bread and drinks from the cup, he brings judgment on himself as he eats and drinks. That is why many of you are sick and weak, and several have died. If we would examine ourselves first, we would not come under God's judgment.[157]

20. Sophocles: Blood Debt

In *Oedipus Tyrannus*, the cause of disease, infertility, and degradation is specifically an unanswered blood debt following a murder. The entire population will suffer until the defilement is purged.

> A plague is on all our host, and thought
> can find no weapon for defence. The fruits
> of the glorious earth grow not; by no birth
> of children do women surmount the pangs
> in which they shriek; and life on life
> mayest thou see sped, like bird on nimble
> wing, aye, swifter than resistless fire, to
> the shore of the western god. . . .
>
> By such deaths, past numbering, the city
> perishes: unpitied, her children lie on the
> ground, spreading pestilence, with none to
> mourn.[158]

This disorder is not to be healed from within. It must be removed or purged for a cure to be effected.

> Phoebus our lord bids us plainly to drive
> out a defiling thing which . . . hath been
> harboured in this land, and not to harbour
> it, so that it cannot be healed.[159]

The murder must be reconciled by very specific human acts of retribution:

> By banishing a man, or by bloodshed in
> quittance of bloodshed, since it is that
> blood which brings the tempest on our
> city.[160]

In this context, divine retribution is also seen as the underlying force:

For our health (with the gods' help) shall
be made certain—or our ruin.[161]

Yet even here the role of the afflicted person's
behavior and attitude in healing is considered:

Give a loyal welcome to my words and
minister to thine own disease [so that]
thou mayest hope to find succor and relief
from woes.[162]

In this play, human misdeed leads to human
suffering and disease. Physicians cannot cure it;
the whole social structure and the individual
woes will only be relieved when a prescribed action is taken and an evil expelled. Like an ab-
scess, the societal affliction must be addressed and
opened up. Only after identifying an evil and
rendering a specific ritual therapy can healing
take place. Ritual therapies are still valued;
though less drastic, they are still generally applied
sometimes without a clear understanding of the
total effect. Antipyretics (aspirin, acetaminophen) are ritually taken for fever. In some mild
cases when the fever is not too high, the fever
may be part of a protective mechanism—a natural response to leukocytic pyrogens that could ac-
tivate other mechanisms of protection. The
function of fever as a host response, if any, is not
completely understood. We treat the symptom of
fever to relieve the febrile person as a comforting
rite, not knowing for sure if the benefit of this
relief is a greater good than the effect of the fever
itself on the battle between the host and the in-
vader in the case of an infectious agent. Recent
studies have shown that some antipyretic therapy
(in children susceptible to Reye's syndrome, for
example) may be harmful and even contraindi-
cated. As we learn more and more about mechanisms of disease, some ritual treatments may be
corroborated as valuable; others may be vitiated
as actually harmful and discarded or replaced.

21. Herodotus: Preventive Purging and Hippocrates Revisited

erodotus reports that other cultures also treated disease as a consequence of sin:

"If a Persian has the leprosy he is not allowed to enter into a city or to have any dealings with the other Persians; he must, they say, have sinned against the sun."[163]

But the disease here is not just a generic plague used as a tool to bring about justice; it is a specific malady connected with the sun. The sun was only one of a number of Persian gods; what is the connection to leprosy? The ancient world frequently labeled as leprosy what is sometimes called "white leprosy" and is now known as vitiligo. The lesions of this disease are pronounced on skin that is exposed to the sun, and they are very sun-sensitive.

Similarly, Herodotus's report of epidemic hysteria is within the realm of the natural and not the supernatural. It swept specifically the guilty Agyllans when they viewed the unburied corpses of prisoners of war whom they had massacred.

Afterwards, when . . . men of the district of Agylla passed by the spot where the murdered Phocaeans lay, their bodies became distorted, or they were seized with palsy, or they lost the use of some of their limbs. On this the people . . . sent to Delphi to ask the oracle how they might expiate their sin.[164]

This reaction is not unlike the conversion hysteria that causes blindness in soldiers who, having narrowly escaped themselves, see comrades destroyed before their eyes.

Herodotus also records, with approabation, the Babylonian approach to the treatment of disease. Expiation of sin does not even enter into their approach, nor do professional physicians. Rather, medicine is seen as an observational science practiced as a matter of public health:

> They have no physicians, but when a man
> is ill, they lay him in the public square,
> and the passers-by come up to him, and if
> they have ever had his disease themselves
> or have known any one who has suffered
> from it, they give him advice,
> recommending him to do whatever they
> found good in their own case, or in the
> case known to them.[165]

Of course, in the case of a contagious infectious disease, this approach is liable to produce more disease than it cures! But a similar networking approach to treatment has emerged in the homosexual community in its efforts to educate its members about the acquired immunodeficiency syndrome (AIDS). Similar networking education efforts also have developed for patients with systemic lupus erythematosus, arthritis, multiple sclerosis, and ostomies, to name a few.

Perhaps most interesting is Herodotus's assessment of Egyptian medical practices. Curiously, his report indicates an inversion of the relationship of disease to religion, for the extraordinary (for the time) sanitation and hygiene practices of the Egyptians were not for the sake of health but only for religious purity:

> They drink out of brazen cups, which they
> scour every day; there is no exception to
> this practice. . . . They practice
> circumcision for the sake of cleanliness.
> . . . The priests shave their bodies every
> other day that no lice or other impure
> thing may adhere to them.[166]

The Egyptians echoed the relationship between diet and health discussed previously. However, instead of carefully regulating their diet, they chose to practice a rather radical lavage:

> For three successive days in each month
> . . . they purge the body by means of
> emetics and clysters, which is done out of
> regard for their health, since they have a
> persuasion that every disease to which men
> are liable is occasioned by the substances
> on which they feed.[167]

Herodotus does praise the Egyptians for their remarkable good health but disagrees about the basis for it. Dismissing ritual purity and preventive purging, he brings basic Hippocratic tenets to the fore. It is through no action of theirs that the Egyptians are a healthy lot.

[The Egyptians are] . . . next to the Libyans, the healthiest people in the world—an effect of their climate, in my opinion, which has no sudden changes. Diseases almost always attack men when they are exposed to a change, and never more than during changes of the weather.[168]

This point of view is in agreement with the previously discussed Hippocratic perspective on temperature and seasonality in human disease. With changes come stress and alterations in the environment (molds and pollens, for example), both of which can contribute to human illnesses. If you do not believe in the significance of rapid changes in the weather, especially rapidly falling atmospheric pressure, talk to someone with rheumatoid arthritis or ankylosing spondylitis!

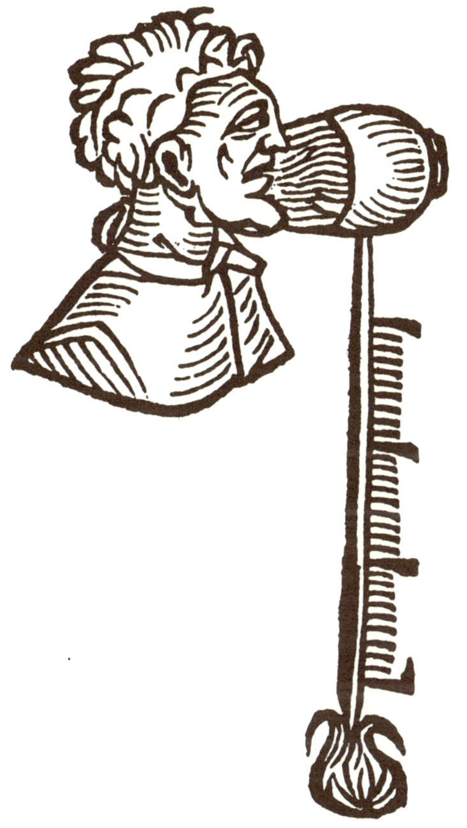

Early thermometers tracked the response of internal heat to external changes.

22. Plato: Disorderly Excesses and Therapeutic Nihilism

Just as in other commentaries, Plato, in writing about diseases and their causes, emphasizes the salutary effect of proportion and balance and the deleterious effect of excess and disproportion. The body politic and the body human are similarly affected.

> The excessive increase of anything often causes a reaction in the opposite direction; and this is the case not only in the seasons and in vegetable and animal life but above all in forms of government.[169]

In the human body, disproportions can lead to severe problems:

> Take the analogy of the body: The evil of the body is a disease which wastes and reduces and annihilates the body.[170]

Plato, in commenting on the stress of the elements on military personnel, emphasizes the same elements widely taught in the Hippocratic school.

> Amid the many changes of water and also of food, of summer heat and winter cold . . . [our warrior athletes] must not be liable to break down in health.[171]

Injurious agents themselves do not cause disease by being nearby; they must interact with the person:

> Even the badness of food, whether staleness, decomposition, or any other bad quality, when confined to the actual food, is not supposed to destroy the body: although, if the badness of food

communicates corruption to the body,
then we should say that the body has been
destroyed by a corruption of itself, which is
disease.[172]

Once again in this listing of causes of disease, we hear about the four fundamental natures and their excess or deficit:

Now everyone can see whence diseases
arise. There are four natures out of which
the body is compacted, earth and fire and
water and air, and the unnatural excess or
defect of these, or the change of any of
them from its own natural place into
another, or—since there are more kinds
than one of fire and of the other
elements—the assumption by any of these
of a wrong kind, or any similar irregularity,
produces disorders and diseases; for when
any of them is produced or changed in a
manner contrary to nature, the parts
which were previously cool grow warm,
and those which were dry become moist,
and the light become heavy and the heavy
light; all sorts of changes occur.[173]

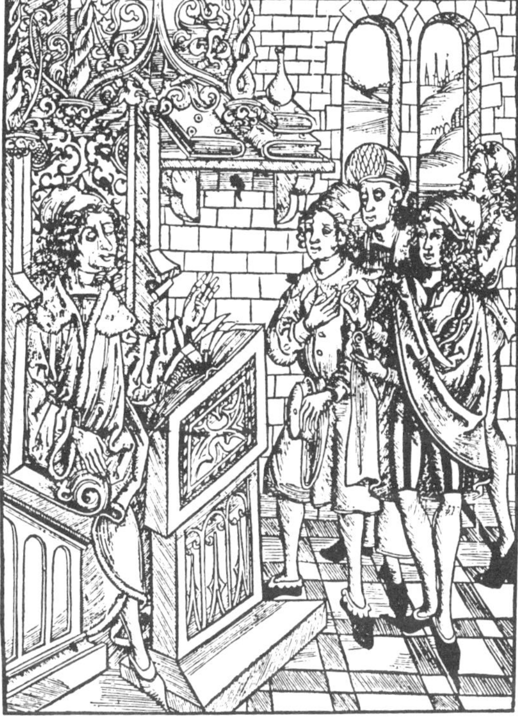

If order results in health, then disorder in disease:

> When each process takes place in this
> [natural] order, health commonly results;
> when in the opposite order, disease. For
> when the flesh becomes decomposed and
> sends back the wasting substance into the
> veins, then an over-supply of blood of
> diverse kinds, mingling with air in the
> veins, having variegated colors and bitter
> properties, as well as acid and saline
> qualities, contains all sorts of bile and
> serum and phlegm. For all things go the
> wrong way, and having become corrupted,
> first they taint the blood itself, and then
> ceasing to give nourishment to the body
> they are carried along the veins in all
> directions, no longer preserving the order
> of their natural courses, but at war with
> themselves, because they receive no good
> from one another, and are hostile to the
> abiding constitution of the body, which
> they corrupt and dissolve.[174]

We would interpret the biochemistry and physiology differently but would agree that alterations in tissues and organs are reflected in the blood constituents and that accumulations of various metabolic products from one particular organ (for example, unconjugated bilirubin and the developing central nervous system, urea, and platelet function) can and do harm others.

In case there are questions about what happens to medical school faculty who deal with disputations and skeptical students, Plato offers the following:

> When teaching or disputing in private or
> in public and strifes and controversies arise
> [an impassioned soul] inflames and
> dissolves the composite frame of man and
> introduces rheums; and the nature of this
> phenomenon is not understood by most
> professors of medicine, who ascribe it to
> the opposite of the real cause.[175]

Once again, the medical school faculties have it just backward.

> Doctors must not rush to treat unless
> treatment is indicated; diseases should
> sometimes be allowed to run their natural
> course. The question of effectiveness of
> therapeutic intervention has always been
> with us.

Diseases unless they are very dangerous should not be irritated by medicines, since every form of disease is in a manner akin to the living being, whose complex frame has an appointed term of life. For not the whole race only, but each individual—barring inevitable accidents—comes into the world having a fixed span, and the triangles in us are originally framed with power to last for a certain time, beyond which no man can prolong his life. And this holds also of the constitution of diseases; if anyone regardless of the appointed time tries to subdue them by medicine, he only aggravates and multiplies them. Wherefore we ought always to manage them by regimen, as far as a man can spare the time, and not provoke a disagreeable enemy by medicines.[176]

Control of diabetic ketoacidosis is necessary and life-saving; yet it is still to be demonstrated that long-term control of hyperglycemia in diabetics diminishes small-vessel changes.

23. Aristotle: Blood and Fat

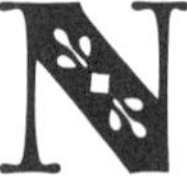Now we write about and discuss consumption coagulopathy and the many conditions in which it occurs. Aristotle's theories sound fanciful to us but the observations held a kernel of truth.

> The case of blood is similar: cold dries and so solidifies it. . . . Diseased blood will not solidify . . . for such blood is of the nature of serum and that is phlegm and water, the nature of the animal having failed to get the better of it and digest it.[177]

Urinary tract stones are commonly discussed in medical historical literature, perhaps because the obstructing object was so real and permanent that there could not be much debate about its role in the patient's disease.

The bladder also is of the nature of membrane, but of membrane peculiar in kind, for it is extensile. . . . In addition to the normal liquid excretion, it passes at times dry excretion also, which turns into stones in the case of sufferers from that malady. Indeed instances have been known of concretions in the bladder so shaped as closely to resemble cockleshells.[178]

Blood and bleeding have long been topics of great medical interest; their function and properties have long been subjects of medical writing:

> In sanguineous animals blood is the most universal and the most indispensable part. . . . When flesh is lacerated, blood exudes, if the animal be alive and unless

the flesh be gangrened. Blood in a healthy condition is naturally sweet to the taste, and red in color; blood that deteriorates from natural decay or from disease is more or less black.[179]

Phlebotomy is only rarely performed therapeutically now, but in prior eras it could be a severe problem for the patient. Now we sometimes remove large amounts of blood from patients for diagnostic studies; only in the rarest of circumstances is this of detriment to the patient. Aristotle reported accurately:

If blood be removed or if it escape in any considerable quantity, animals fall into a faint or swoon; if it be removed or if it escape in an exceedingly large quantity, they die.[180]

The following observations, on the other hand, now have drastically different interpretations as to cause and effect and pathological relationships:

If the blood get diseased, hemorrhoids may ensue in the nostril or at the anus, or the veins may become varicose. Blood, if it corrupt in the body, has a tendency to

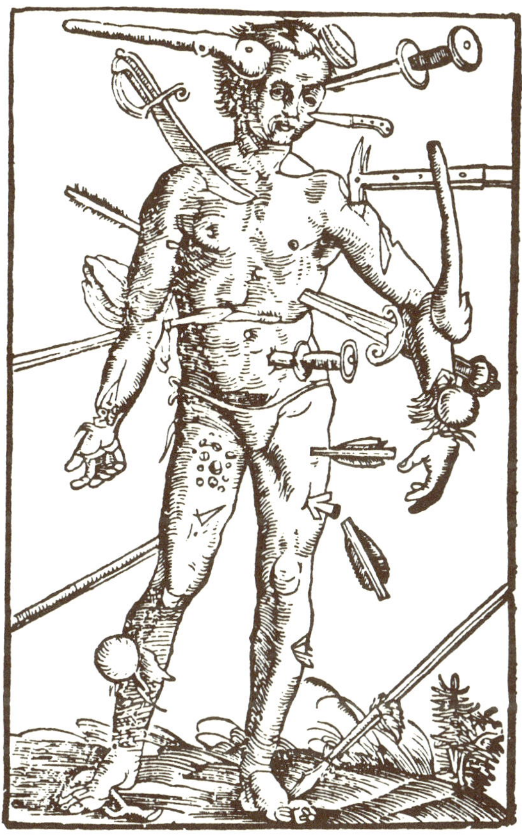

A *sanguineous illustration of bloodletting sites.*

turn into pus, and pus may turn into a solid concretion.[181]

Aristotle, like Thomas Aquinas and modern cardiologists to follow, perceived the ill effects of excessive saturated animal fats in the diet, although without specifying the nature of the injury. Hippocrates, as we shall see, also paid a great deal of attention to the role of diet in disease.

Both lard and suet when present in moderate amount are beneficial; for they contribute health and strength, while they are no hindrance to sensation. But when they are present in great excess, they are injurious and destructive.[182]

24. Hippocrates: Diet, Climate, and Cold Phlegm

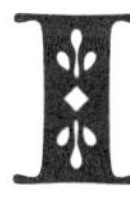In *On Ancient Medicine*, we find a rather simplified explanation of the cause of disease and death:

[Men] suffered much from [a] . . . strong and brutish diet swallowing things which were raw, unmixed, and possessing great strength, they become exposed to strong pains and diseases, and thereby to early deaths.[183]

We also learn that

no one disease is either more divine or more human than another, but that all are alike divine, for that each has its own natural cause.[184]

In determining the best outcome for the patient, physicians then and now need to know their limitations and regulate their actions upon the disease. Hippocrates tells us:

I would give great praise to the physician whose mistakes are small, for perfect accuracy is seldom to be seen, since many physicians seem to me to be in the same plight as bad pilots, who, if they commit mistakes while conducting the ship in a calm do not expose themselves, but when a storm and violent hurricane overtake them, they then, from their ignorance and mistakes, are discovered to be what they are, by all men, namely, in losing their ship. And thus bad and commonplace physicians, when they treat men who have no serious illness, in which case one may commit great mistakes without producing any formidable mischief (and such complaints occur much more frequently to men than dangerous ones): under these circumstances, when they commit mistakes, they do not expose themselves to ordinary men; but when they fall in with a great, a strong, and a dangerous disease, then their mistakes and want of skill are made apparent to all. Their punishment is not far off, but is swift in overtaking both the one and the other.[185]

Every student of medicine strives to learn how to detect the difference between greater and lesser diseases and, as pointed out in the Hippocratic text, must know when the former is the case. This discrimination is important not only because with the graver conditions is the tolerance for error less, but also because in these disorders the intrinsic resilience of the human organism is sometimes reduced drastically and is much less a factor in favor of the doctor and the patient than is the case with lesser afflictions.

Dietary changes, mild and drastic alike, as illustrated in the following citations played an inordinate role in ancient medical thinking.

There are certain persons who cannot readily change their diet with impunity; and if they make any alteration in it for one day, or even for a part of a day, are greatly injured thereby.[186]

Let him eat wheat, such as it is supplied from the thrashing-floor, raw and unprepared, with raw meat, and let him drink water. By using such a diet I know that he will suffer much and severely, for he will experience pains, his body will become weak, and his bowels deranged, and he will not subsist long. . . . [Such] articles of food, those which are unsuitable and hurtful to man when administered, every one is either bitter, or intensely so or saltish or acid, or something else intense and strong, and therefore we are disordered by them in like manner as we are by the secretions of the body.[187]

The Hippocratic advice about the physician acquainting himself or herself with both form and function by learning anatomy and physiology as foundation sciences for medicine is carried on in western medicine:

One ought also to know what diseases arise in man from the powers, and what from the structures. . . . By powers I mean intense and strong juices; and by structures, whatever conformations there are in man. For some are hollow, and from broad contracted into narrow; some expanded, some hard and round, some broad and suspended, some stretched, some long, some dense, some rare and succulent, some spongy and of loose texture.[188]

The following fanciful interpretations of congestion and edema might be of interest to the medical student struggling to learn pathology:

The bladder, the head, the uterus in a woman; these parts which are hollow and expanded are most likely to receive any humidity flowing into them, but cannot attract it in like manner. Those parts which are solid and round could not attract a humidity, nor receive it when it flows to them, for it would glide past, and find no place of rest on them. But spongy and rare parts, such as the spleen, the

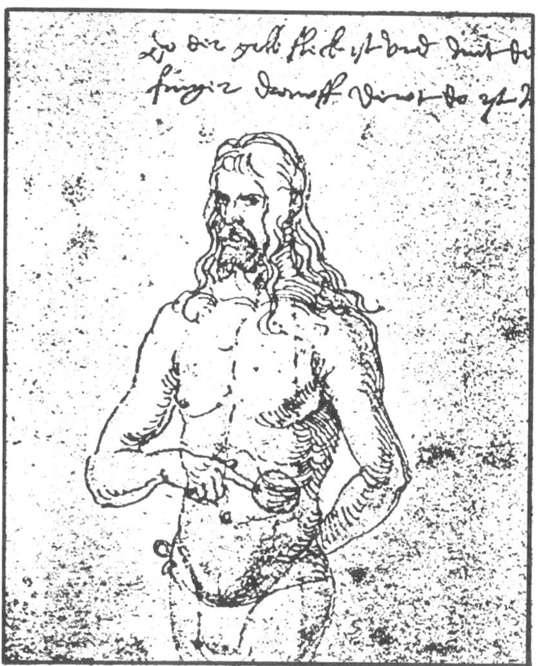

A *patient's sketch locates pain . . . perhaps a splenic tumor.*

lungs, and the breasts, drink up especially the juices around them, and become hardened and enlarged by the accession of juices. . . . When [the spleen] drinks up and receives a fluid into itself, the hollow and lax parts of it are filled, even the small interstices; and, instead of being rare and soft, it becomes hard and dense, and it can neither digest nor discharge its contents.[189]

The Hippocratic school emphasized general environmental hazards, such as the type of water supply consumed, in the causation of kidney or bladder stones:

Men become affected with the stone, and are seized with diseases of the kidneys, strangury, sciatica, and become ruptured, when they drink all sorts of waters, and those from great rivers into which other rivulets run, or from a lake into which many streams of all sorts flow and such as are brought from a considerable distance.[190]

We now look for what possible metabolic stress or disease might be affecting each urinary tract stone patient. Instead of evaluating the general nature of the water supply, we look to the serum calcium level or the parathyroid endocrine status of each patient. Even if we were to concede that the water supply were important in helping to determine disease patterns, in *On Regimen in Acute Disease* we are again reminded of the importance of the disequilibrium brought about by rapid change. In the broader context, abrupt change in water supply may be more important than the nature of any given water supply.

One may derive information from the regimen of persons in good health what things are proper; for if it appears that there is a great difference whether the diet be so and so, in other respects, but more especially in the changes, how can it be otherwise in diseases, and more especially in the most acute? But it is well ascertained that even a faulty diet of food and drink steadily persevered in, is safer in the main as regards health than if one suddenly change it to another.[191]

Change is easier to implement in health but is always potentially dangerous:

The greatest changes as to those things which regard our constitutions and habits are most especially concerned in the production of diseases, for it is impossible to produce unseasonably a great emptying of the vessels by abstinence, or to administer food while diseases are at their acme, or when inflammation prevails; nor, on the whole, to make a great change either one way or another with impunity.[192]

Some diseases discussed in these writings are recognized as specific lesions that we see today (pharyngeal abscesses, for example). Our current explanation, though, is quite different from the ancient:

> Quinsy takes place when a copious and viscid defluxion from the head, in the season of winter or spring, flows into the jugular veins, and when from their large size they attract a greater defluxion; and when owing to the defluxion being of a cold and viscid nature it becomes enfarcted, obstructing the passages of the respiration and of the blood, coagulates the surrounding blood, and renders it motionless and stationary, it being naturally cold and disposed to obstructions. Hence they are seized with convulsive suffocation, the tongue turning livid, assuming a rounded shape, and being vent owing to the veins which are seated below the tongue.[193]

Then, as now, not maintaining an airway had serious consequences. In *On Epidemics*, we read about some of the more serious effects of infection by *Streptococcus pyogenes* that are occasionally still seen, although rarely, because of antimicrobic therapy.

> Early in spring, along with the prevailing cold, there were many cases of erysipelas. . . . They were of a malignant nature, and proved fatal to many; many had sore-throat and loss of speech. There were many cases of ardent fever, phrensy, aphthous affections of the mouth, tumors on the genital organs; of ophthalmia, anthrax, disorder of the bowels, anorexia, with thirst and without it; of disordered urine, large in quantity and bad in quality;

of persons affected with coma for a long time, and then falling into a state of insomnolency.[194]

Current understanding of seizure disorders does not endorse the conclusions presented here in *Sacred Disease;* yet the modern reader may well enjoy the historical perspective on this common malady that was also so important to the writers of the New Testament:

> When a defluxion of cold phlegm takes place on the lungs and heart, the blood is chilled, and the veins, being violently chilled, palpitate in the lungs and heart, and the heart palpitates, so that from this necessity asthma and orthopnea supervene. For it does not receive the spirits as much breath as he needs until the defluxion of phlegm be mastered, and being heated is distributed to the veins, then it ceases from its palpitation and difficulty of breathing, and this takes place as soon as it obtains an abundant supply. . . . If the defluxions be more condensed, the epileptic attacks will be more frequent, but otherwise if it be rarer. Such are the symptoms when the defluxion is upon the lungs and heart; but if it be upon the bowels, the person is attacked with diarrhea.[195]

Here the description attempts to go beyond demonology and details the results of loss of sphincter control.

25. Galen: Causes of Edema

In *On Natural Faculties*, we read explanations of peripheral edema and other conditions that would not be accepted today but give us background on the commonly used terms of nutrition and assimilation and other disease states:

Nutrition . . . an assimilation of that which nourishes to that which receives nourishment. And in order that this may come about, we must assume a preliminary process of adhesion, and for that, again, one of presentation. . . . The so-called white [leprosy] shows the difference between assimilation and adhesion, in the same way that the kind of dropsy which some people call anasarca clearly distinguishes presentation from adhesion. For, of course, the genesis of such a dropsy does not come about as do some of the conditions of atrophy and wasting, from an insufficient supply of moisture; the flesh is obviously moist enough—in fact it is thoroughly saturated—and each of the solid parts of the body is in a similar condition. While, however, the nutriment conveyed to the part does undergo presentation, it is still too watery, and is not properly transformed into a juice, nor has it acquired that viscous and agglutinative quality which results from the operation of innate heart; therefore, adhesion cannot come about, since, owing to this abundance of thin, crude liquid, the pabulum runs off and easily slips away from the solid parts of the body. In white [leprosy], again, there is adhesion of the nutriment but no real assimilation. From this it is clear that what I have just said is correct, namely, that in that part which is to be nourished there must first occur presentation, next adhesion, and finally assimilation proper.[196]

Now, we would associate edema with many pathophysiological states; however cirrhosis and severe anemia are still among them:

> [Some] imagine that dropsy is . . . always [caused] by induration of the liver. . . . We have observed dropsy produced by hemorrhoids . . . through immoderate bleeding . . . and by violent bleeding from the womb.[197]

Now hemorrhoids, in some cases, are known to be secondary to liver disease and portal hypertension; no doubt some of the more severe cases are still associated with palpable induration of the liver. Though associated with liver disease, hemorrhoids are known not to cause it. Galen tells us that:

> A kind of dropsy . . . is brought about by an excessive chilling of the whole constitution . . . which is the primary reason for the occurrence of dropsy, results from a failure of blood-production, very much like diarrhea which follows imperfect digestion of food . . . . In this kind of dropsy neither the liver nor any viscus becomes indurated.[198]

Perhaps we would best relate this sort of edema to renal disease with hypoproteinemia, since no visceral organs are enlarged.

Galen may be talking about gastrointestinal hemorrhage or melena along with diarrhea causing the effects to be more serious for the patient:

> Hippocrates says, "Dysentery is a fatal condition if it proceeds from black bile"; while that proceeding from the yellow bile is by no means deadly, and most people recover from it; this proves how much more pernicious and acrid in its potentialities is black than yellow bile.[199]

We still think of the reticuloendothelial system in the spleen as a sort of filter but no longer associate splenomegaly with evil humors or consider the spleen itself as a cause of disease by inducing humoral imbalances:

The spleen is a viscus . . . which cleanses
the blood . . . . In those cases in which
the spleen is large and is increasing from
internal suppuration, it destroys the body
and fills it with evil humors.[200]

Nor do we think of it as a sop for dark or black
bile pigments that regulate the hue and viscosity
of the blood.

Thus, just as the kidneys, whose function
it is to attract the urine, do this badly
when they are out of order, so also the
spleen, which has in itself a native power
of attracting an atrabiliary quality, if it
ever happens to be weak, must necessarily
exercise this attraction badly, with the
result that the blood becomes thicker and
darker.[201]

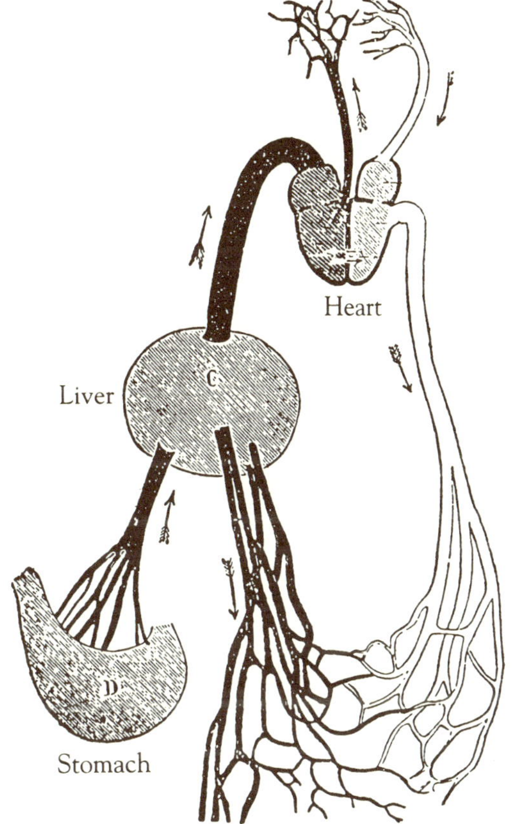

*Galen's theory of the
motion of the blood.*

26. Plotinus: Cause from Cure?

In the *Second Ennead*, we learn that physicians and magicians are alike in at least one respect when they try to explain diseases to their patients.

> Magicians . . . can never persuade the intelligent that disease arises otherwise than from such causes as overstrain, excess, deficiency; in a word, some variation whether from within or from without.[202]

Some very intelligent persons to this day keep a version of the ancient popular faith alive in their persistent beliefs in the scientifically unsubstantiated roles of vitamins and other mysterious and poorly defined dietary constituents—in excess of deficiency—as well as other vagaries of life in either protecting health or promoting disease.

Examples are legion; one only need look into a modern health food store: alfalfa tablets, zinc supplements, and megadose regimens for trace vitamins, etc.

Plotinus points out that, in contrast to some folk wisdom theories, diseases have causes. Evil spirits and other mysteries have a lesser role in this presentation on the cause of disease:

> [Nonetheless they claim] the nature of illness is indicated by its very cure. A motion, a medicine, the letting of blood, and the disease shifts down and away; sometimes scantiness of nourishment restores the system: presumably the spiritual power gets hungry or is debilitated by the purge. Either this spirit makes a hasty exit or it remains within. If it stays,

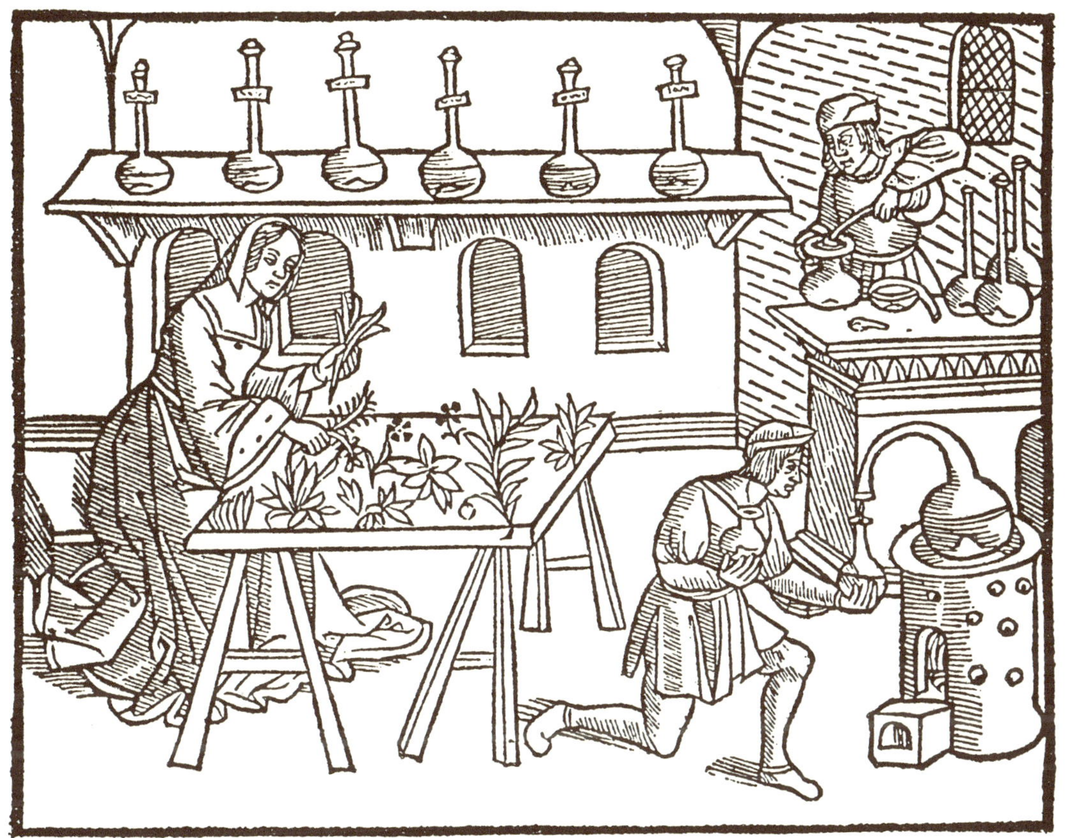

Among folk remedies there is no shortage of real and imaginary cures.

how does the disease disappear, with the cause still present? If it quits the place, what has driven it out? Has anything happened to it? Are we to suppose it throve on the disease? In that case the disease existed as something distinct from the spirit-power. Then again, if it steps in where no cause of sickness exists why should there be anything else but illness? If there must be such a cause, the spirit is unnecessary: that cause is sufficient to produce that fever. As for the notion, that just when the cause presents itself the watchful spirit leaps to incorporate itself with it, this is simply amusing.[203]

Physicians must deal in some positive or constructive way with their patients' beliefs, of whatever sort, in order to be more effective healers. Unsound as some popular wisdoms may be to a scientifically trained physician, the doctor may find it quite beneficial to the healing process to empathize with the patient's beliefs when explaining the modern theory of his particular disease to him. Plotinus' sarcasm or ironic approach is not likely to be well received in this context!

27. Aquinas: Gluttons Beware!

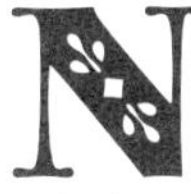Not a whole lot in medicine changed between Galen and Aquinas. In *Summa Theologica*, we learn that familial traits were appreciated, but the distinction between genetics and environment had not been made:

Defects of the body are transmitted from parent to child; thus a leper may beget a leper, or a gouty man may be the father of a gouty son, on account of some seminal corruption, although this corruption is not leprosy or gout.[204]

The constitution remains most important, and disequilibrium is an underlying cause of disease:

[There is a kind] of habit [that] is the disposition of a complex nature, according to which that nature is well or ill disposed to something, chiefly when such a disposition has become like a second nature, as in the case of sickness or health. . . . Bodily sickness is a disordered disposition of the body, by reason of the destruction of that equilibrium which is essential to health.[205]

Omission and commission apply to the body as well as the soul:

Bodily sickness is partly a privation, in so far as it denotes the destruction of the equilibrium of health, and partly something positive, namely the very humours that are disposed in a disordered way.[206]

Temperature variations and extremes continue to be important:

Various species of sickness proceed from different causes, for example from excessive heat or cold, or from a lesion in the lung or liver.[207]

And degrees of illness can be discerned and explained:

Sickness of the body, even sickness of the same species, has not an equal cause in all; for instance if a fever be caused by corruption of the bile, the corruption may be greater or lesser, and nearer to, or further from a vital principle.[208]

The idea of contagion was well comprehended:

Those corruptions especially are said to be infectious which are of such a nature as to be transmitted from one subject to another; hence contagious diseases, such as leprosy and mange and the like, are said to be infectious.[209]

Aquinas held hypernutrition in general as deleterious, as Aristotle had done on the ill effects of eating too much animal fat: "Some sicken and die through eating too much."[210] Perhaps they both were hinting at a contributing cause of a now common disease that is seriously aggravated by overeating and a diet high in animal fat—the major cause of death in modern North America—arteriosclerotic cardiovascular disease.

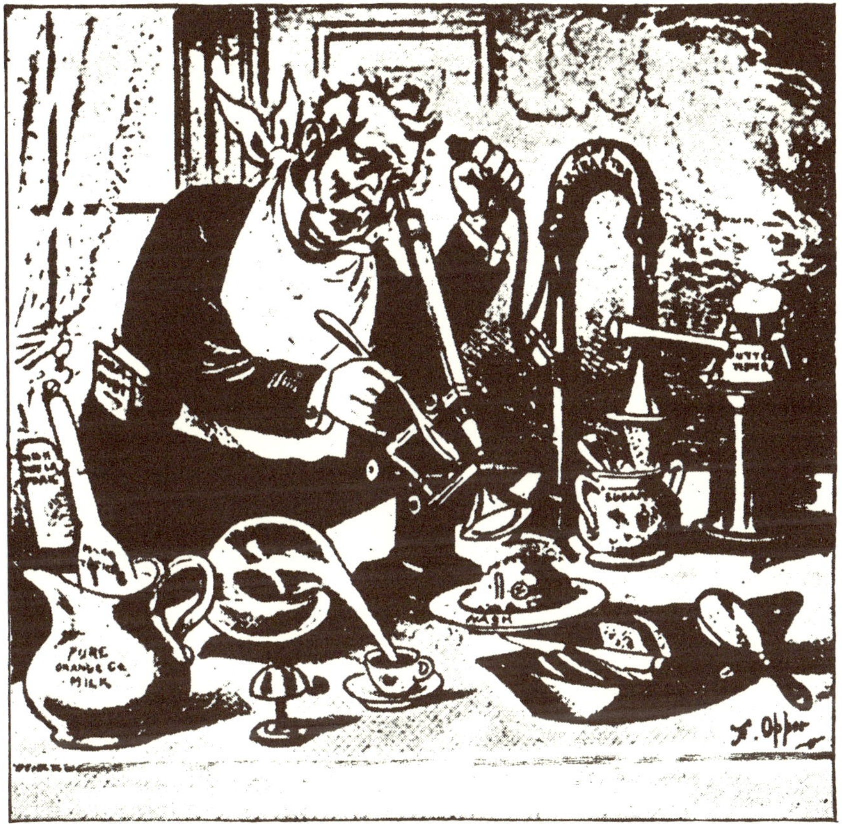

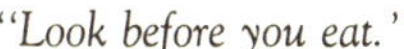

"Look before you eat."

28. Chaucer and Montaigne: The Doctor and His Critics

In *The Canterbury Tales* by now familiar elements are repeated, and dicta of medical practice dating back to the Hippocratic era appear again.

With us there was a doctor of physic;
In all this world was none like him to pick
For he was grounded in astronomy.
He often kept a patient from the pall
By horoscopes and magic natural
Well could he tell the fortune ascendent
Within the houses for his sick patient.
He knew the cause of every malady,
Were it of hot or cold, of moist or dry,
And where engendered, and of what
  humour;
He was a very good practitioner.
The cause being known, down to the
  deepest root,
Anon he gave to the sick man his boot.
Ready he was, with his apothecaries,
To send him drugs and all electuaries;
By mutual aid much gold they'd always
  won—
Their friendship was a thing not new
  begun.[211]

The affinity between physician and gold continues to be one that plagues the relationship between the medical profession and the public in one form or another.

Montaigne, in his *Essays*, does a great deal of editorializing about medicine and its practitioners. Along with that of other observers, his work predicts some aspects of what is to be learned about genetics:

What a wonderful thing it is that the drop

of seed from which we are produced should
carry in itself the impression not only of
the bodily form, but even of the thoughts
and inclinations of our fathers![212]

This concept he further personalizes in his own
life experience:

'Tis to be believed that I derive this
infirmity from my father, for he died
wonderfully tormented with a great stone
in his bladder.[213]

His attitude toward physicians is rather skeptical and embittered, even to the point of accus-
ing doctors of provoking ailments so as to
enhance their practices:

I see no people so soon sick, and so long
before they are well, as those who take
much Physic; their very health is altered
and corrupted by their frequent
prescriptions. Physicians are not content to
deal only with the sick, but they will
moreover corrupt health itself, for fear
men should at any time escape their
authority.[214]

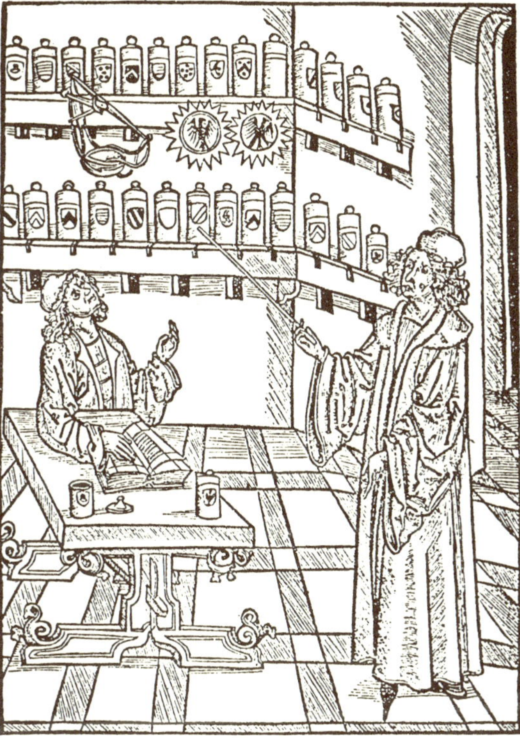

*A physician choosing
"electuaries," drugs that by
another name taste more
sweet.*

In our current concern about the various issues involved in determining drugs to be both safe and effective, it would, perhaps, be well to consider the following:

The violent gripings and contest betwixt the drug and disease are ever to our loss, since the combat is fought within ourselves, and that the drug is an assistant not to be trusted, being in its own nature an enemy to our health and by trouble having only access into our condition. Let it alone a little: the general order of things that takes care of fleas and moles also takes care of men, if they will have the same patience that fleas and moles have, to leave it to itself.[215]

The healing power of nature is a theme that recurs time and again through the ages.

Montaigne offers a couple of comments that truly reflect his attitude toward the medical profession:

Order a purge for your brain, it will there be much better employed than upon your stomach.[216]

[Physicians have this advantage] that the sun gives light to their success and the earth covers their failures.[217]

29. Harvey: Cacodemons and Cacochemy

In *Motion of the Heart*, Harvey reiterates the age old concept of a central fire within the living organism:

The circulation is [a] matter both of convenience and necessity . . . since all living things are warm, all dying things cold, there must be . . . [a place where] . . . the native fire is stored and preserved; whence heat and life are dispensed to the parts as from a fountain head[218]

He continues his emphasis on the importance of his favored humor and the heart:

The heart is the principle of life. . . . The blood, therefore, is required to have motion, and indeed such a motion that it should return again to the heart; for sent to the extreme parts of the body far from its fountain, as Aristole says, and without motion, it would become congealed. . . .

The blood, therefore become thick or congealed by the cold of the extreme and outward parts, and robbed of its spirits just as in the dead, it was imperative that from its fount and origin, it should again receive heat and spirits, and all else requisite to its preservation—that, by returning, it should be renovated and restored. . . .

Unless the heart were truly that fountain where life and heat are restored to the refrigerated fluid and whence new blood, warm, imbued with spirits, being sent out by the arteries, that which has become

cooled and effete is forced on, and all the
particles recover their heat which was
failing, and their vital stimulus well-nigh
exhausted.[219]

And he offers us a simplified presentation of the
then prevalent viewpoints on disease, echoing
earlier writings of Plotinus and Galen:

> The schoolmen . . . hold some diseases to
> be owing to a Cacodemon or evil spirit, as
> there are others that are due to a
> cacochemy or defective assimilation.[220]

The teaching in medical schools, influenced
by Avicenna, still emphasized various spirits
coursing via different routes to cause disease; perhaps Plotinus would consider the medical faculty
so teaching to be more magicians than physicians:

> Medical schools admit three kinds of
> spirits: the natural spirits flowing through
> the veins, the vital spirits through the
> arteries, and the animal spirits through the
> nerves.[221]

His recurring point of view, though, is to return
to the overwhelming importance of the circulatory system to anchor his own interpretation of
human disease:

> It seems that the spirits which flow by the
> veins or the arteries are not distinct from
> the blood, any more than the flame of a
> lamp is distinct from the inflammable
> vapour that is on fire; in short, that the
> blood and these spirits signify one and the
> same thing, though different—like
> generous wine and its spirit; for as wine,
> when it has lost all its spirit, is no longer
> wine, but a vapid liquor or vinegar; so
> blood without spirit is not blood, but
> something else—clot or cruor.[222]

In spite of this emphasis he has not totally abandoned the miasmic theory; in *On Animal Generation* we read:

> Medical men observe contagious diseases,
> such as leprosy, lues venera, plague,
> phthisis, to creep through the ranks of
> mortal men, and by mere extrinsic contact
> to excite diseases similar to themselves in
> other bodies; nay, contact is not necessary;
> a mere halitus or miasm suffices, and that

at a distance and by an inanimate medium, and with nothing sensibly altered.[223]

He also points out that blood, particularly as a transport medium, is involved in disease as well as health.

> Nor is the blood the author of life only, but, according to its diversities, the cause of health and disease likewise: so that poisons, which come from without, such as poisoned wounds, unless they infect the blood, occasion no mischief. Life and death, therefore, flow for us from the same spring.[224]

That which refreshes can also poison.

Harvey also appreciated genetic predispositions:

> And this too is a remarkable fact, that virtues and vices, marks and moles, and even particular dispositions to disease are transmitted by parents to their offspring; and that while some inherit in this way, all do not.[225]

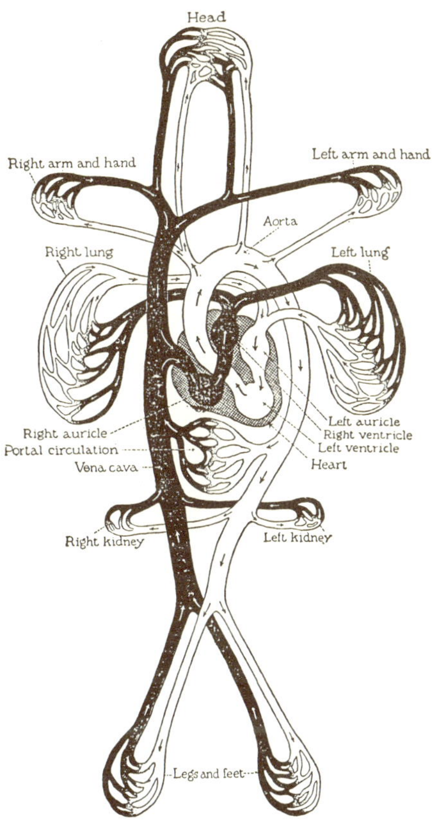

Harvey's theory of the true course of the circulation of the blood, by experimentation.

He did not know about sympathetic and parasympathetic nervous impulses and neurosecretory granules but had a great appreciation for how the cardiovascular system functions:

> When the heart, for example, is affected with palpitation, tremor, lipothymia, syncope, and with great variety in the extent, rapidity, and order or rhythm of its pulsations, we do not hesitate to ascribe these to morbific causes implicating, deranging its sensation. For whatever by its divers movements strives against irritations and troubles must necessarily be endowed with sensation.[226]

He did, it should be mentioned, pay some tribute to what were then considered to be the lesser systems:

> The stomach and bowels, disturbed by the presence of vitiated humours, are affected with ructus, flatus, vomiting, and diarrhoea; and as it lies not in our power either to provoke or to restrain their motions, neither are we aware of any sensation dependent on the brain which should arouse the parts in question to motions of the kind.[227]

Two hundred years later, the fundamentally modern cellular basis for disease was developed and first expounded in the Institute of Pathology in Berlin.

30. Virchow: The Little Giant of Pathology

This diminutive physician-scientist ar-cheologist, and social activist, probably more than any other person brought modern experimental medicine into the day-to-day practice of physicians. His concept of the cell as the center of all pathological changes was critical in reorganizing our thinking on the mechanisms of disease. His meticulous approach to observation of microscopic tissue changes is still with us in the 1980s.

Virchow's work, starting shortly after Müeller's discovery of the animal cell and Schwann's work on the importance of nucleated animal cells, detailed the importance of the cell as the basic element in life and disease. He maintained and consolidated the modern belief that all cells come from cells (*omnis cellulae e cellula*).[228] In 1858, his ideas and early work were collected in a series of lectures for practicing physicians in Berlin at the Institute of Pathology, which had been built especially for him. They were subsequently published as his pivotal book, *Cellular Pathology*. In it, his goal was to offer:

> A view of the cellular nature of all vital processes, both physiological and pathological, animal and vegetable, so as distinctly to set forth what even the people have long been dimly conscious of, namely the unity of life in all organized beings in opposition to the one-sided humoral . . . tendencies which have been transmitted from the mythical days of antiquity to our own times.[229]

His emphasis was on cells and cellular mechanisms of disease, as manifested in anatomical tissue changes seen with the light microscope. His influence in initiating an orderly study of tissues in various diseases by systematic autopsies and by rigorously examining histologic sections was crucial in allowing development of a coherent, organized system for classifying and studying diseases. His basic approach is still applied. He emphasized the "application of histology to pathology to obtain a recognition of the fact that the cell is really the ultimate morphological element in which there is any manifestation of life."[230]

In his antihumoral posture he was breaking with long tradition. He stated that he respected tradition but also maintained "that even in this there is a certain limit. Too great respect is a real fault, for it favors confusion."[231] Proper, precise, clarifying terminology waas very important for him. Some of the ideas and terms he developed or elaborated importantly upon include: parenchymatous inflammation, thrombosis and embolization, leukemia, ichorrhaemia (icterus or jaundice), osteoid and mucous tissue, caseous and amyloid metamorphosis, and substitution of tissues (metaplasia). He declared inflammation to be definite (a controversial point in his era):

I cannot help allowing inflammation to be a definite form in which pathological processes display themselves, although I am unable to admit its claims to be regarded as an entity.[232]

We still consider the cellular aspects of inflammatory processes as important, even diagnostic, manifestations of certain diseases in tissue biopsies. Virchow added a concept regarding cancer as a new growth or neoplastic process that we still value. He stated, "I must . . . maintain epithelioma [squamous carcinoma] a heteroplastic, malignant new-formation (cancroid)."[233] Cancer is still understood as new tissue arising from host cells, then proliferating in and sometimes invading throughout the host.

Virchow repudiated the then popular humoral theory. He emphasized the cell and light microscopically visible tissue alterations in diseases rather than speculations about humors, vapors, and spirits. We now have gone beyond and into the cell and are studying cell surface and other receptors, hormones, mediators, and molecules still not clearly defined in modern efforts to understand homeostasis and mechanisms of disease.

The effort now is in investigating subcellular and molecular structure and function, but Virchow's basic approach to developing careful systems of studying organs, tissues, and cells morphologically to elucidate understandings of disease is still applied in modern pathology.

His view of disease and the microscopic tissue changes that accompany it included the concept of cell territories. One can imagine territorially oriented cellular citizens coming into conflict in disease in much the same way that Plato and Hobbes discussed civil war as an analogy for disease. Pathologists in the 1980s talk about autoimmune diseases such as lupus erythematosus being, in a way, the consequence of such a civil war between lymphocytes and other cells in various organs.

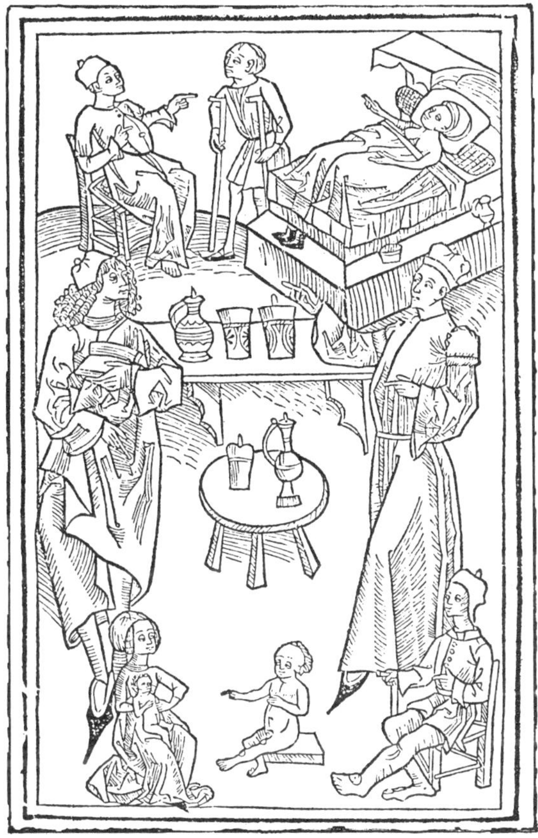

Conclusion

This work has been prepared particularly for the present or future physician but also for general readers to demonstrate what selected eminent past students of nature have said about knowledge of human disease and its applications in medical practice. By philosophical analysis, collected observations, and records of individual case histories, we have seen how certain insights into aspects of doctor-patient relationships and the medical art have persisted through the centuries. Many of the most venerated customs of medicine have very deep cultural roots; the works collected here expose some of them for the modern reader and allow a closer look.

Medicine continues to work with, and enhance the natural processes of, healing and endeavors to discover new ways of applying phenomena of nature to aid healing and maintain health. Strict control of all vital endogenous homeostatic and healing mechanisms has not been attained and is not likely to be achieved soon. Whether such control is truly possible or desirable is debatable. We know that modern science will continue to allow us closer and closer views of the intricacies of cellular and subcellular functions. We shall be inundated with raw data and basic observations. Whether we shall be able to digest this information, assimilate it as knowledge, and apply it appropriately in individual patient contexts and still maintain the nurturing and gentle aspects of our healing tradition is a very important question. Doctors of medicine must know about diseases, their classifications, and their human contexts—general and individual—in order to diagnose, prognose, and accurately measure the effects of their therapeutic regimens. Past insights will certainly aid today's students in addressing evolving questions about the nature of diseases and the best approaches for the doctor and patient in coping with them in their manifold and changing forms.

Certain current ideas about human disease have been reviewed and discussed in this work; we have seen that some—if not many—are not new or even recent. From studying this compendium, the reader can appreciate selected insights from different eras into medicine and the healing arts and see not only how they are especially relevant in our present approaches to dealing with the personal concerns and individual circumstances of each patient but also how they still apply to our way of thinking about the cause and nature of disease.

References

1. Plato *Charmides* 156.
2. Plato *Charmides* 156.
3. Plato *The Republic* 3.403.
4. Plato *Charmides* 157.
5. Plato *The Republic* 3.404.
6. Plato *The Republic* 3.405.
7. Plato *The Republic* 3.406.
8. Plato *The Republic* 3.407.
9. Plato *The Republic* 3.406.
10. Hippocrates *On Ancient Medicine* 13.
11. Hippocrates *On Ancient Medicine* 14.
12. Hippocrates *On Ancient Medicine* 19.
13. Hippocrates *On Ancient Medicine* 9.
14. Aristotle *History of Animals* 3.19.
15. Aristotle *History of Animals* 7.1.
16. Aristotle *On the Parts of Animals* 2.7.
17. Aristotle *On the Parts of Animals* 2.7.
18. Aristotle *On the Parts of Animals* 4.2.
19. Aristotle *On the Parts of Animals* 4.2.
20. Aristotle *Rhetoric* 1.5.
21. Aristotle *Rhetoric* 2.5.
22. Aristotle *Rhetoric* 2.5.
23. Aristotle *Rhetoric* 2.5.
24. Galen *On the Natural Faculties* 2.8.
25. Galen *On the Natural Faculties* 2.8.
26. Galen *On the Natural Faculties* 2.8.
27. Galen *On the Natural Faculties* 2.8.
28. Galen *On the Natural Faculties* 2.9.
29. Galen *On the Natural Faculties* 2.9.
30. Galen *On the Natural Faculties* 2.9.

31. Galen *On the Natural Faculties* 2.9.

32. Galen *On the Natural Faculties* 1.12.

33. Galen *On the Natural Faculties* 1.12.

34. Galen *On the Natural Faculties* 2.9.

35. Galen *On the Natural Faculties* 2.9.

36. Galen *On the Natural Faculties* 2.9.

37. Galen *On the Natural Faculties* 2.9.

38. Harvey *An Anatomical Disquisition on the Motion of the Heart and Blood in Animals*, chap. 15.

39. Harvey *Motion of the Heart* 15.

40. Harvey *Anatomical Exercises on the Generation of Animals* 71.

41. Harvey *Anatomical Exercises on the Generation of Animals* 71.

42. Aquinas *Treatise on Habits* 73.3.

43. Plato *The Republic* 4.444.

44. Plato *The Republic* 10.556.

45. Plato *Timaeus* 82.

46. Plato *Timaeus* 84.

47. Plato *Timaeus* 84.

48. Plato *Timaeus* 84.

49. Plato *Symposium* 186.

50. Plato *Symposium* 186.

51. Hobbes *Leviathan* 2.29.

52. Hobbes *Leviathan* 2.29.

53. Hobbes *Leviathan* 2.29.

54. Hobbes *Leviathan* 2.29.

55. Aristotle *On the Generation of Animals* 5.4.

56. Aristotle *On the Generation of Animals* 5.4.

57. Aristotle *On the Generation of Animals* 5.4.

58. Aristotle *On the Generation of Animals* 5.4.

59. Aristotle *On the Generation of Animals* 5.4.

60. Aristotle *Nicomachean Ethics* 2.2.

61. Aristotle *Nicomachean Ethics* 2.2.

62. Hippocrates *On Ancient Medicine* 14.

63. Hippocrates *On Ancient Medicine* 14.

64. Hippocrates *On Ancient Medicine* 14.

65. Hippocrates *On Ancient Medicine* 14.

66. Galen *On the Natural Faculties* 2.8.

67. Galen *On the Natural Faculties* 2.8.

68. Galen *On the Natural Faculties* 2.8.

69. Galen *On the Natural Faculties* 2.8.

70. *Avicenna's Tract on Cardiac Drugs and Essays on Arab Cardiotherapy.* New Delhi: Institute of History of Medicine and Medical Research, 1963, p. 11.

71. *Avicenna's Tract on Cardiac Drugs and Essays on Arab Cardiotherapy,* p. 17.

72. *Avicenna's Tract on Cardiac Drugs and Essays on Arab Cardiotherapy,* p. 23.

73. Maimonides: Regimen sanitatis. *Transactions of the American Philosophical Society,* New Series 54(4):16, 1964.

74. Maimonides: Regimen sanitatis, p. 16.

75. Maimonides: Regimen sanitatis, p. 17.

76. Maimonides: Regimen sanitatis, p. 17.

77. Maimonides: Regimen sanitatis, p. 17.

78. Maimonides: Regimen sanitatis, p. 19.

79. Maimonides: Regimen sanitatis, p. 21.

80. Maimonides: Regimen sanitatis, p. 21.

81. Maimonides: Regimen sanitatis, p. 21.

82. Maimonides: Regimen sanitatis, p. 27.

83. Maimonides: Regimen sanitatis, p. 28.

84. Maimonides: Regimen sanitatis, p. 30.

85. Harvey *The First Anatomical Disquisition on the Circulation of the Blood,* chap. 1.

86. Harvey *Circulation of the Blood,* chap. 1.

87. Harvey *Circulation of the Blood,* chap. 1.

88. Plato *Timaeus* 81.

89. Plato *Timaeus* 83.

90. Plato *Timaeus* 83.

91. Plato *Timaeus* 84.

92. Plato *Timaeus* 85.

93. Hippocrates *On Airs, Waters, and Places* 3.

94. Hippocrates *On Airs, Waters, and Places* 5.

95. Hippocrates *On Airs, Waters, and Places* 6.

96. Hippocrates *On Airs, Waters, and Places* 7.

97. Hippocrates *On Regimen in Acute Diseases* 2.

98. Hippocrates *Of the Epidemics* 3.1.

99. Hippocrates *Of the Epidemics* 3.2.

100. Hippocrates *Of the Epidemics* 3.2.

101. Hippocrates *On Airs, Waters, and Places* 1.

102. Hippocrates *On Injuries of the Head* 4–8.

103. Hippocrates *On Fractures* 31.

104. Hippocrates *On Articulations* 61.

105. Hippocrates *On Articulations* 61.

106. Hippocrates *On Articulations* 62.

107. Hippocrates *Aphorisms* 3.5.

108. Hippocrates *Aphorisms* 3.9.

109. Hippocrates *Aphorisms* 3.15, 16.

110. Hippocrates *Aphorisms* 3.19–23.

111. Leviticus 13.2–5.

112. Leviticus 13.9–14.

113. Aristotle *On the Generation of Animals* 9.326.

114. Leviticus 15.2–6.

115. Leviticus 15.31.

116. Langmuir A.D., et al.: The Thucydides syndrome: A new hypothesis for the cause of the plague of Athens. *N. Engl. J. Med.* 313:1027–1030, 1985.

117. Thucydides *History of the Peloponnesian War* 2.7.47–49.

118. Hippocrates *Book of Prognostics* 1.

119. Hippocrates *Book of Prognostics* 1.

120. Hippocrates *Book of Prognostics* 2.

121. Hippocrates *Book of Prognostics* 3.

122. Hippocrates *Book of Prognostics* 4.

123. Hippocrates *Book of Prognostics* 5.

124. Hippocrates *Book of Prognostics* 8.

125. Hippocrates *Book of Prognostics* 9.

126. Hippocrates *Book of Prognostics* 11.

127. Hippocrates *Book of Prognostics* 12.

128. Hippocrates *Book of Prognostics* 13.

129. Hippocrates *Book of Prognostics* 14.

130. Hippocrates *Book of Prognostics* 17.

131. Hippocrates *Book of Prognostics* 19.

132. Hippocrates *Book of Prognostics* 21.

133. Hippocrates *Book of Prognostics* 22.

134. Hippocrates *Book of Prognostics* 23.

135. Hippocrates *Book of Prognostics* 25.

136. Hippocrates *On Regimen in Acute Diseases* 9.

137. Hippocrates *On Regimen in Acute Diseases* 9.

138. Hippocrates *On Regimen in Acute Diseases* 15.

139. Hippocrates *On Regimen in Acute Diseases* 22.

140. Hippocrates *On Injuries of the Head* 19.

141. Hippocrates *On Injuries of the Head* 19.

142. Lucretius *On the Nature of Things* 3.459.

143. Lucretius *On the Nature of Things* 3.487.

144. Lucretius *On the Nature of Things* 6.1110.

145. Lucretius *On the Nature of Things* 6.1138.

146. Leviticus 26.16.

147. Numbers 12.9–12.

148. Numbers 16.46–49.

149. Deuteronomy 28.20–22.

150. Deuteronomy 28.27.

151. Deuteronomy 28.28.

152. Deuteronomy 28.28.

153. II Maccabees 9.5–6.

154. II Maccabees 9.8–9.

155. Matthew 9.32.

156. Matthew 17.15–18.

157. I Corinthians 11.29–32.

158. Sophocles *Oedipus the King* 170–180.

159. Sophocles *Oedipus the King* 94–96.

160. Sophocles *Oedipus the King* 100–102.

161. Sophocles *Oedipus the King* 145–146.

162. Sophocles *Oedipus the King* 216–218.

163. Herodotus *The History* 1.139.

164. Herodotus *The History* 1.139.

165. Herodotus *The History* 1.197.

166. Herodotus *The History* 2.37.

167. Herodotus *The History* 2.77.

168. Herodotus *The History* 2.77.

169. Plato *The Republic* 8.563.

170. Plato *The Republic* 10.609.

171. Plato *The Republic* 3.404.

172. Plato *The Republic* 3.609.

173. Plato *Timaeus* 81, 82.

174. Plato *Timaeus* 82, 83.

175. Plato *Timaeus* 88.

176. Plato *Timaeus* 89.

177. Aristotle *Meteorology* 4.7.384a25–30.

178. Aristotle *On the History of Animals* 3.15.519b.

179. Aristotle *On the History of Animals* 3.19.520b10–21.

180. Aristotle *On the History of Animals* 3.19.521a10.

181. Aristotle *On the History of Animals* 3.19.521a19–20.

182. Aristotle *On the Parts of Animals* 2.5.651a36.

183. Hippocrates *On Ancient Medicine* 3.

184. Hippocrates *On Airs, Waters, and Places* 22.

185. Hippocrates *On Ancient Medicine* 9.

186. Hippocrates *On Ancient Medicine* 10.

187. Hippocrates *On Ancient Medicine* 13–15.

188. Hippocrates *On Ancient Medicine* 22.

189. Hippocrates *On Ancient Medicine* 22.

190. Hippocrates *On Airs, Waters, and Places* 9.

191. Hippocrates *On Regimen in Acute Diseases* 9.

192. Hippocrates *On Regimen in Acute Diseases* 9.

193. Hippocrates *On Regimen in Acute Diseases*, Appendix, para. 6.

194. Hippocrates *Of the Epidemics* 3.3.3.

195. Hippocrates *On the Sacred Disease* 9.

196. Galen *On the Natural Faculties* 1.11.

197. Galen *On the Natural Faculties* 2.8.

198. Galen *On the Natural Faculties* 2.8.

199. Galen *On the Natural Faculties* 2.9.

200. Galen *On the Natural Faculties* 2.9.

201. Galen *On the Natural Faculties* 2.9.

202. Plotinus *Second Ennead* 9.14.

203. Plotinus *Second Ennead* 9.14.

204. Aquinas *Summa Theologica* 2:1, q. 81, art. 1.

205. Aquinas *Summa Theologica* 2:1, q. 82, art. 1.

206. Aquinas *Summa Theologica* 2:1, q. 82, art. 1.

207. Aquinas *Summa Theologica* 2:1, q. 82, art. 2.

208. Aquinas *Summa Theologica* 2:1, q. 82, art. 4.

209. Aquinas *Summa Theologica* 2:1, q. 83, art. 4.

210. Aquinas *Summa Theologica* 2:1, q. 85, art. 5.

211. Chaucer *Canterbury Tales*, Prologue 411–428.

212. Montaigne *The Essays* 2.37.

213. Montaigne *The Essays* 2.37.

214. Montaigne *The Essays* 2.37.

215. Montaigne *The Essays* 2.37.

216. Montaigne *The Essays* 2.37.

217. Montaigne *The Essays* 2.37.

218. Harvey *An Anatomical Disquisition on the Motion of the Heart and Blood in Animals*, chap. 15.

219. Harvey *The First Anatomical Disquisition on the Circulation of the Blood in Animals*, disq. 2, point 3.

220. Harvey *The First Anatomical Disquisition on the Circulation of the Blood in Animals*, disq. 2, point 3.

221. Harvey *The First Anatomical Disquisition on the Circulation of the Blood in Animals*, disq. 2, point 3.

222. Harvey *The First Anatomical Disquisition on the Circulation of the Blood in Animals*, disq. 2, point 3.

223. Harvey *Anatomical Exercises on the Generation of Animals* 49.

224. Harvey *Anatomical Exercises on the Generation of Animals* 52.

225. Harvey *Anatomical Exercises on the Generation of Animals* 57.

226. Harvey *Anatomical Exercises on the Generation of Animals* 57.

227. Harvey *Anatomical Exercises on the Generation of Animals* 57.

228. Virchow R.: *Cellular Pathology, as Based on Physiological and Pathological Histology.* Philadelphia: P. Blakiston Sons & Co., 1858, p. 54.

229. Virchow R.: *Cellular Pathology,* p. v.

230. Virchow R.: *Cellular Pathology,* p. 29.

231. Virchow R.: *Cellular Pathology,* p. 239.

232. Virchow R.: *Cellular Pathology,* p. vii.

233. Virchow R.: *Cellular Pathology,* p. vii.

Index

Figure Acknowledgments

51 From *A History of Medicine*, by Arturo Castiglioni. New York: Alfred A. Knopf, 1947. Reprinted by kind permission of Laura Castiglioni Luzzatto Giuliani.

52 The changing characteristics of illustrations of the four temperaments are discussed in Raymond Klibansky, Edwin Panofsky, and Fritz Saxl, *Saturn and Melancholy: Studies in the History of Natural Philosophy, Religion and Art*. London: T. Nelson & Sons; New York: Basic Books, 1964. Reprint by Kraus-Thompson, Mendeln, Liechtenstein, 1979, now Millwood, N.Y., 1979. Reprinted by kind permission of Professor Klibansky.

57 From *A History of Medicine*, by Arturo Castiglioni. New York: Alfred A. Knopf, 1947. Reprinted by kind permission of Laura Castiglioni Luzzatto Giuliani.

65 From *Early Books on Medicine, Natural Sciences and Alchemy* (Catalogue of Books). Lugano, Italy: L'Art Ancien SA, 1926–1928.

68, 73 75, 81 From *A History of Medicine*, by Arturo Castiglioni. New York: Alfred A. Knopf, 1947. Reprinted by kind permission of Laura Castiglioni Luzzatto Giuliani.

86 From *A History of Medicine*, by Brian Inglis. Cleveland: World Publishing, 1965.

91 From *A Short History of Medicine*, by Charles Joseph Singer. Oxford: Oxford University Press, 1962.

97 Reprinted by permission of the Bettmann Archive, New York City.

99 From *A History of Medicine*, by Arturo Castiglioni. New York: Alfred A. Knopf, 1947. Reprinted by kind permission of Laura Castiglioni Luzzatto Giuliani.

103 From *History of Medicine*, by Fielding H. Garrison. Philadelphia: W.B. Saunders Co., 1929.

107 From *A History of Medicine*, by Arturo Castiglioni. Sketch by Albrecht

Durer. New York: Alfred A. Knopf, 1947. Reprinted by kind permission of Laura Castiglioni Luzzatto Giuliani.

113 From *Behind the Doctor*, by Logan Clendening. Illustrated by James E. Bodrero and Ruth Harris Bohan. Copyright 1933 by Alfred A. Knopf and renewed by Mrs. Alfred B. Clark. Reprinted by permission of the publisher.

115 From *Early Books on Medicine, Natural Sciences and Alchemy* (Catalogue of Books). Lugano, Italy: L'Art Ancien SA, 1926–1928.

119, 121 From *A History of Medicine*, by Arturo Castiglioni. New York: Alfred A. Knopf, 1947. Reprinted by kind permission of Laura Castiglioni Luzzatto Giuliani.

125 From *The Human Body*, fourth edition, by Logan Clendening. Revised by W.C. Shepard. Illustrated by Dale Beronius. Copyright 1945 by Alfred A. Knopf and renewed by Mrs. Alfred B. Clark. Reprinted by permission of the publisher.

129 From *Nature Disclosed* (Catalogue of Selected Books in the John Crerar Collection of Rare Books in the History of Science and Medicine), by Anthea Waleson. Chicago: University of Chicago, 1983. Reprinted by permission of the University of Chicago Library.

158 From *Dictionaire des illustrateurs*, by Marcus Osterwalder. Engraving by Adolfo Bongini, between 1908 and 1925. Paris: Hubschmid & Bouret, 1983.

Text Acknowledgments

Permission to reprint passages from texts by the following writers has been granted by the following individuals or institutions and is gratefully acknowledged.

Aristotle, Chaucer, Plato—Oxford University Press, Oxford, England.

Aquinas—Benziger, Bruce & Glencoe, Encino, California.

Avicenna—Institute of History of Medicine and Medical Research, New Delhi.

Galen—Harvard University Press and the Loeb Classical Library, Cambridge, Mass.

Harvey, Hippocrates, Hobbes, Lucretius, Rabelais, Sophocles—Encyclopaedia Britannica, Inc., Chicago.

Herodotus—J.M. Dent & Sons, Ltd., London.

Maimonides—American Philosophical Society, Philadelphia.

Montaigne—G. Bell & Sons, Ltd., London.

Plotinus—Sir Ernest R. Debenham, Dorset, England.

Thucydides—E.P. Dutton & Co., New York.

All biblical quotations are from the *Good News Bible*, published by the American Bible Society, New York, in 1976.

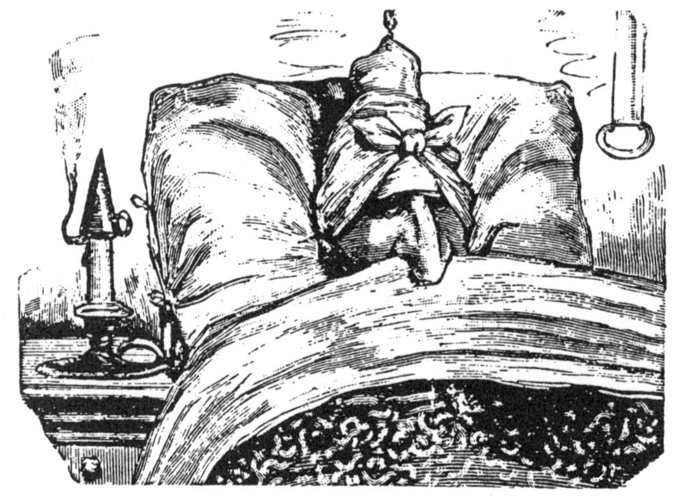

FIN